Student Workbook for Fundamentals of Nursing

Carol Taylor, R.N., M.S.N.
Carol A. Lillis, R.N., M.S.N.
Priscilla LeMone, R.N., M.S.N.

Student Workbook prepared by
Nu-Vision, Inc.
Kansas City, Missouri

J..B. Lippincott Company

Philadelphia

London Mexico City New York
St. Louis Sau Paulo Sidney

Student Workbook for Fundamentals of Nursing

Printed in the United States of America. For information address J. B. Lippincott Company, East Washington Square, Philadelphia, PA 19105.

6 5 4 3 2 1

ISBN 0-397-54752-8

Contributing Authors

Nu-Vision, Inc.
Carolyn H. Brose, R.N., Ed.D., President
Paula S. Cokingtin, R.N., M.S.N., Vice-President
Kathy D. Robinson, R.N., M.S.N., Vice-President

Jan Carter, R.N., M.N., O.C.N.
Consultant,
Nu-Vision, Inc.
Kansas City, Missouri

Carol J. Green, R.N., M.N.
Instructor Department of Nursing
Johnson County Community College
Overland Park, Kansas

Evelyn Hutchison, R.N., M.S.
Professor Emeritus
Central Missouri State University
Warrensburg, Missouri

Deborah J. Kenny, R.N., M.S.N., Ed.M.
Instructor
University of Kansas
Kansas City, Kansas

Penny Marshall, R.N., M.S.N.
Instructor Department of Nursing
Johnson County Community College
Overland Park, Kansas

Ardyce Plumlee, R.N., M.N.
Assistant Professor
University of Kansas
Kansas City, Kansas

Cheryl L. Stover, R.N., M.S.N.
Assistant Professor
Central Missouri State University
Warrensburg, Missouri

Mary E. Young, R.N., M.A.N.
Professor Emeritus
Central Missouri State University
Warrensburg, Missouri

Judith Wilkinson, R.N.C, M.A., M.S.
Instructor Department of Nursing
Johnson County Community College
Overland Park, Kansas

Dina Wilson, R.N., M.S.
Assistant Professor
University of Kansas
Kansas City, Kansas

Table of Contents

Unit V

Roles Basic to Nursing Practice

Unit VI

Actions Basic to Nursing Practice

Unit VII

Promoting Healthy Physiologic Responses

Unit VIII

Promoting Healthy Psychosocial Responses

Unit IX

Promoting Optimal Health in Special Situations

Unit I
The Nurse: Foundations for Nursing Practice

The four chapters which comprise Unit I introduce the concepts of professional nursing, health-illness, and the health care system in society. The learner explores what it means to be an emerging profession and nursing's role as a provider of care. An introduction to nursing theory is given in chapter four; chapters five and six provide a basis for understanding ethical and legal implications of nursing actions and relationships.

Chapter 1
Introduction to Nursing

Chapter 1 of Fundamentals of Nursing (Taylor, 1988) introduces the learner to the historical context of the emerging profession of nursing. The organizational structure of the profession, educational preparation, and contemporary roles of nursing are presented. After studying this chapter and completing the associated workbook exercises the student should be able to

- Define key terms used in the chapter.
- Describe the historical background, the definitions, and the professional status of nursing.
- Identify the aims of nursing, including nursing activities necessary to promote wellness and prevent illness.
- Describe the various levels of educational preparation and offerings in nursing.
- Discuss the impact on nursing practice of nursing organizations, standards of nursing practice, nurse practice acts, and the nursing process.
- Identify current trends and issues in nursing.

Key Terms Chapter 1

You will want to become familiar with the meaning of the following key terms used in this chapter.

continuing education
dependent nursing actions
independent nursing actions
in-service education
interdependent nursing actions
licensure
nurse practice act
profession
standards

Contributions of Florence Nightingale

Florence Nightingale, the "Lady with a Lamp," challenged prejudices against women and had an indisputable impact on nursing and health care during the 19th century.

List 5 contributions of Miss Nightingale.

1. ______________________________
2. ______________________________
3. ______________________________
4. ______________________________
5. ______________________________

6. Why were Miss Nightingale's contributions so unique for her time in history?

____
____
____
____
____

History of Nursing

Place one word in each blank to complete the sentence.

7. During the early Christian period visiting of the sick and afflicted was first organized by a group of women called ______________________.
8. In _______ (year) Miss Nightingale was born in Florence, Italy to a wealthy English family.
9. In the United States, schools of nursing were organized within hospitals and were based more on an _____________ model rather than on an educational model.

The Art of Nursing

Nursing has been defined in many ways but there are essential elements present in most thoughtful perspectives. In your own words, expand on the following short definitions.

10. Nursing is **caring** ______________________________
____
11. Nursing is **sharing** ______________________________
____

12. Nursing is **touching** ____________________

13. Nursing is **feeling** ____________________

14. Nursing is **listening** ____________________

15. Nursing is **accepting** ____________________

16. Nursing is **believing** ____________________

Key Terms: Match

Match the terms with the appropriate definitions.

Terms:

a. dependent nursing actions
b. nursing
c. in-service education
d. licensure
e. interdependent nursing actions
f. nursing education
g. independent nursing actions
h. holistic health care
i. continuing education
j. nurse practice act
k. nursing process
l. professional standards

Definitions:

17. ____ The education of L.P.N.'s and R.N.'s.
18. ____ Lays the foundation for the practice of professional nursing.
19. ____ A method of organizing and giving nursing care.
20. ____ Laws regulating nursing.
21. ____ Collaboration with other members of the health care team.
22. ____ The education and training of employees by an institution.
23. ____ Response to health care team members.
24. ____ Planned learning experiences beyond basic nursing education.
25. ____ Activities based on assessment, knowledge, and judgment.
26. ____ Became more formalized with the advent of Christianity.
27. ____ Incorporates physical, psychosocial, and spiritual dimensions.
28. ____ Legal right to practice nursing.

Crossword puzzle

Use the clues below to solve the crossword puzzle.

DOWN

1. Nurse practice acts
2. The focus of nursing is _____.
4. Proposed A.D. nursing education programs
5. Nursing's response to society
6. Step four of the nursing procsss
8. Basis of post WWII nursing schools
9. Licensed practical nurse
11. Wellness-illness
13. American Nurses' Associaton
15. "Nutrix"
17. Step two of nursing process
19. National League for Nursing
21. First school of nursing
22. Core of nursing
25. Focus of nursing care

ACROSS

3. First step of nursing process
7. Nursing aims to restore
10. Professional characteristic
12. May be dependent, interdependent, or independent
14. Number of steps in the nursing process
15. Established first schools of nursing
16. Growing client population
18. Canadian Nurses' Association
20. First international organization of professional women
23. Facilitated by nursing
24. National Council Licensure Exam
26. Nursing organization open to non-nurses
27. Final step of nursing process
28. Preparation for specialty practice
29. Never exists in isolation
30. Defines activities of nurses

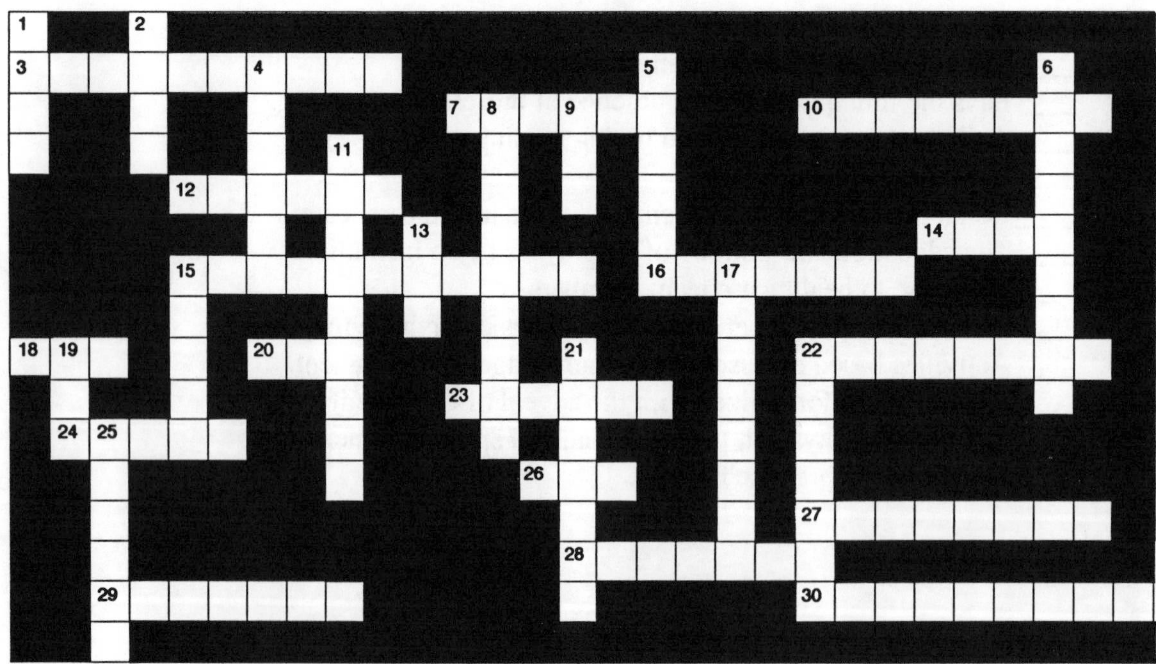

Nursing Organization Acronyms

Write out the names of the organizations associated with the acronyms listed below.

29. ANA ______
30. ICN ______
31. NLN ______
32. NSNA ______
33. CNA ______

Expanded Nursing Roles

Differentiate between the nursing roles listed below by completing the table.

TITLE	Education/Preparation	Role Description
Example: *Nurse Researcher*	*advanced degree*	*conducts research relevant to nursing practice and education*
34. Nurse Midwife	a.	a.
35. Nurse Practitioner	b.	b.
36. Nurse Anesthetist	c.	c.

Additional Enrichment Activities

1. Obtain a copy of the nurse practice act for your state. Examine/read in order to be familiar with the law in your state.
2. Explore the various educational programs for graduate nurses in your community. Are they accredited by the National League for Nursing?
3. Locate the addresses of national headquarters for the ANA, NLN, and ICN. How would membership in each organization benefit you?
4. List the **independent** nursing actions which nurses on the unit where you work are implementing. Contrast this list with the dependent nursing actions.
5. Plan a bulletin board display of current newspaper articles and pictures of nursing.
6. Develop a five minute speech and/or slide show about early nursing.

Suggested Readings

American Nurses' Association: Nursing and Social Policy Statement. Kansas City, MO, American Nurses' Association, 1980

Canadian Nurses' Association: A Definition of Nursing Practice: Standards for Nursing Practice. Ottawa, Canadian Nurses' Association, 1980

Characteristics of Baccalaureate Education in Nursing. National League for Nursing, Pub No 15-1758, 1978

Competencies of the Associate Degree Nurse on Entry into Practice. New York, National League for Nursing, Pub No 23-1731, 1978

Donahue MP: Nursing the Finest Art: An Illustrated History. St. Louis, CV Mosby, 1985

Downs F, Brooten D: New Careers in Nursing. New York, New York, Arco Publishing, Inc., 1984

Dolan J: Nursing in Society: A Historical Perspective. Philadelphia, WB Saunders, 1978

Ellis J, Hartley C: Nursing in Today's World: Challenges, Issues, Trends, 3rd ed. Philadelphia, JB Lippincott, 1988

Grippando GM: Nursing Perspectives and Issues. Albany, New York, Delmar Press 1986

International Council of Nurses: 1973 Code for Nurses. Geneva, International Council of Nurses, 1973

Kalish P, Kalish B: The Advance of American Nursing, 2nd ed. Boston, Little, Brown & Co, 1986

Nurses for the future: An AJN Supplement. AJN, 87(12):1593-1657, 1987

Primm PL: Differentiated practice for ADN and BSN prepared nurses. J Professional Nursing 3(4):218-15, 1987

Sullivan TJ et al: Nursing 2020: A study of nursing's future. Nursing Outlook 35(5):233-5, 1987

Chapter 2
Promoting Wellness in Health and Illness

Chapter 2 of Fundamentals of Nursing (Taylor, 1988) is concerned with how the practice of nursing is influenced by both the person receiving care and the nurse giving care. Individualized, holistic care requires that health and illness be understood from the point of view of the client receiving the care.

After studying this chapter and completing the workbook exercises the student should be able to

- Define key terms used in the chapter.
- Define health and illness, using a variety of models.
- Explain the influence of the human dimensions, basic human needs, and self-concept on health and illness status, beliefs, and practices.
- Compare acute illness with chronic illness.
- List the causes of disease and death.
- Summarize the activities of the nurse in promoting wellness and preventing illness, incorporating risk factors, illness behaviors, and the effects of illness on the family.
- Describe the levels of nursing care in promoting wellness and preventing illness.

Key Terms Chapter 2

You will want to become familiar with the meaning of the following key terms used in this chapter.

acute illness
agent-host-environment model
basic human needs
chronic illness
health
health-belief model
health-illness continuum
health-risk appraisal
high-level wellness
illness
primary preventive care
risk factors
secondary preventive care
self concept
tertiary preventive care
wellness

Factors Influencing Health-Illness Status, Beliefs, and Practices

The following questions are related to factors affecting health and illness. Answer the questions in the space provided.

1. List the six human dimensions that influence behaviors of persons receiving health care.
   a. ______________________________
   b. ______________________________
   c. ______________________________
   d. ______________________________
   e. ______________________________
   f. ______________________________
2. A person who becomes ill progresses through the stages of __________, __________, __________.

3. In the space below draw and explain the health-illness continuum.

Health Illness Continuum

4. Where do you fit on the health-illness continuum and why?

____

____

5. List, in descending order, the five leading causes of death in the United States.

1st ______________
2nd ______________
3rd ______________
4th ______________
5th ______________

6. Name six causes of disease.

a. ____
b. ____
c. ____
d. ____
e. ____
f. ____

7. List four acute illnesses.

a. ____
b. ____
c. ____
d. ____

8. List four chronic illnesses.

a. ____
b. ____
c. ____
d. ____

Health, Illness: Key Terms Match

Match the key terms related to health and illness with the appropriate definitions.

Terms:

a. acute illness
b. agent-host-environment model
c. basic human needs
d. chronic illness
e. health
f. health-belief model
g. health-illness continuum
h. health-risk appraisal
i. high-level wellness
j. illness
k. primary preventive care
l. risk factor
m. secondary preventive care
n. self-concept
o. tertiary preventive care
p. wellness

Definitions:

9. ____ The basis for holistic health care.
10. ____ Health is a constantly changing state.
11. ____ Functioning to one's maximum potential.
12. ____ Essential and common to all people.
13. ____ Human dimension that increases chance for illness or injury.
14. ____ A personal concept relative to each individual.
15. ____ A change in structure or function of a person's body or mind.
16. ____ Useful in predicting illness.
17. ____ Based on perceptions.
18. ____ Illness often alters.
19. ____ Permanent alterations or impairment in normal functioning.
20. ____ Following illness, restores to a maximum functioning level.
21. ____ Focus is on prevention of complications or disabilities.
22. ____ A self-limiting illness.
23. ____ Directed towards specific protection against illness.

Levels of Preventive Care

Draw lines to connect the levels of preventive care in Column I with the nursing actions in Column II. Explain the rationale for your choice in Column III.

Column I Level of Preventive Care	Column II Actions	Column III Rationale
	24. Giving medications	24.
	25. Facilitating a support group	25.
Primary	26. Decubitus care	26.
Secondary	27. Teaching self-breast exam	27.
Tertiary	28. Immunizations	28.
	29. Accident prevention education	29.
	30. Dental care	30.
	31. Physical therapy	31.
	32. Range of motion exercises	32.

Case Study

Joan Brown, who is seven months pregnant, is grocery shopping with her two small children. She hasn't really felt well since her husband was killed in an accident six weeks ago. The loss of her mate, the responsibility of her family and financial concerns seem overwhelming. The money set aside for labor and delivery was needed for funeral expenses. Suddenly Joan begins to bleed profusely from the vagina as she enters the check-out area of the store. She is taken to the nearest hospital where she is given immediate attention. As the nurse is doing assessment, Joan begins to sob uncontrollably.

33. List and prioritize Joan Brown's needs using Maslow's hierarchy.

Additional Enrichment Activities

1. Verify three primary, secondary, and tertiary prevention measures being implemented in your community.
2. Complete the Healthstyle Selftest from the National Health Information Clearinghouse (Taylor, p. 27). What changes in lifestyle are indicated by your score?
3. Make a list of your own healthy and not-so-healthy self-care behaviors. Improve two not-so-healthy behaviors in the next 24 hours.

Suggested Readings

Cox CL: The health self-determination index. Nursing Research 34 (3):177-183, 1985

Dunn H: High-Level Wellness. Arlington, VA. RW Teathy, 1961

Hames C, Joseph D: Basic Concepts of Helping: A Wholistic Approach. New York, Appleton-Century-Crofts, 1980

Maslow A: Toward a Psychology of Being, 2nd ed. New York., D Van Nostrand, 1968

Reilly PA et al: Health and life styles: employee wellness. Nursing Administration Quarterly 11(3):29-35, 1987

Computer Assisted Instruction

Wellness-Illness Continuum. Heshi Computing

Chapter 3
The Health-Care System

Chapter 3 of Fundamentals of Nursing (Taylor, 1988) focuses on the rapidly changing health-care system and how the changes impact on nursing care delivery.

After studying the chapter and completing the workbook exercises, the learner should be able to

- Define key terms used in the chapter.
- Discuss the social and economic trends affecting the health-care delivery system.
- Describe the various types of health-care insurance.
- Describe several types of alternative health-care delivery.
- Compare and contrast the various types of health-care agencies.
- Discuss the problems experienced by the health-care system.
- List the services provided by various health-care agencies.

Key Terms Chapter 3

You will want to become familiar with the meaning of the following key terms used in this chapter.

adult day-care centers
ambulatory care centers
continuing-care retirement community
crisis intervention center
diagnostic related groups
extended care facility
governmental agencies
health maintenance organization
home health-care agency
hospice
life-care center
long-term care facilities
Medicaid
Medicare
mutual aid self help groups
preferred provider arrangement
preferred provider organization
prospective payment plan
psychiatric agency
Public Health Service
rehabilitation center
respite care
voluntary health-care agency

Health-Care System: Match

Match the terms with the appropriate definitions.

Definitions:

1. ____ A group plan for financing health care where members pay fixed monthly or annual rates.
2. ____ Predetermined rates assigned to specific health-care procedures.
3. ____ A group plan for financing health-care involving organizations of health-care providers.
4. ____ Same as PPO except can be arranged with individual health-care providers.
5. ____ A plan implemented by the federal government utilizing DRGs in an effort to control rising health-care costs.

Terms:

a. health maintenance organization
b. diagnostic related group
c. preferred provider arrangement
d. preferred provider organization

Definitions:

6. ____ The traditional nursing home or convalescent center.
7. ____ Provide care to the client in the home.
8. ____ Nursing homes where elderly or physically or mentally challenged are cared for.
9. ____ Centers offering independent living units similar to apartments with 24-hour emergency care, as well as intermediate or skilled nursing care when the need arises.
10. ____ Members organize and run self-help groups that offer emotional support and education to their members.

Terms:

a. continuing-care retirement community
b. extended care facility
c. home health-care agency
d. long-term care facility
e. mutual aid self-help group

Definitions:

11. ____ A facility financed by national, state, local or provincial taxes.
12. ____ A federal health agency providing a wide range of services.
13. ____ Non-profit agencies involved in promoting health.
14. ____ An agency that provides counseling, support, and treatment for clients experiencing emotional or behavioral illnesses.

Terms:

a. voluntary health care agency
b. psychiatric agency
c. public health service
d. governmental agencies

Definitions:

15. ____ Provide care to elderly or physically or mentally challenged adults while family members are employed.
16. ____ A walk-in clinic offering the same or similar services as the physician's office.
17. ____ A facility offering independent living units for the handicapped or elderly.
18. ____ A center specializing in returning a client to a pre-illness level of functioning or providing education and training to enable a client to function as independently as possible.
19. ____ A psychiatric center providing immediate assistance, support and guidance for further psychiatric care.

Terms:

a. life-care center
b. adult day-care centers
c. ambulatory care centers
d. crisis intervention center

Health-Care Settings

Complete the crossword puzzle.

Across

1. provides pain relief, symptom management and supportive resources
4. mutual aid self-help group
7. preferred provider arrangement
10. voluntary health-care agencies
12. nursing focus
13. activities of daily living
15. federal insurance program for elderly
16. diagnosis related groups
18. preferred provider organizations
21. National Institute of Health
22. Veteran's Administration
23. provides relief for care-giver
26. avoid to control costs
29. a self-help group dealing with infertility
30. medical doctor

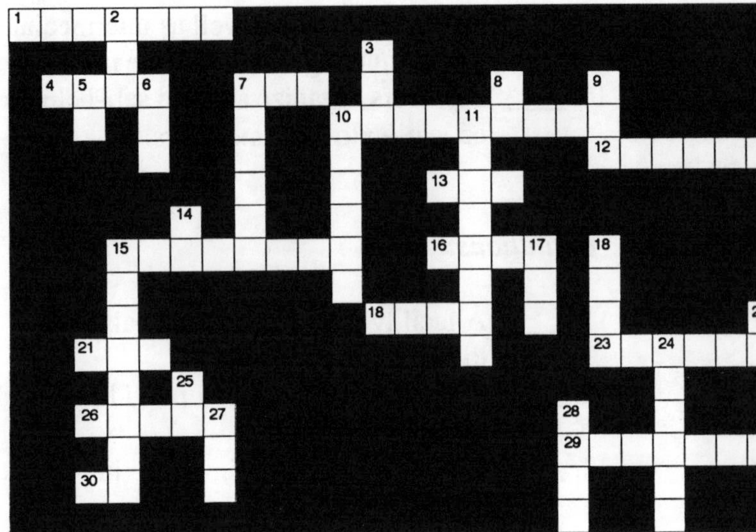

Down

2. Public Health Service
3. health maintenance organization
5. Alcoholics Anonymous
6. home health care
7. hospital financed and operated by local or national government
8. doctor of osteopathy
9. long term care
10. the largest group of professionals within the health care system
11. a non-profit organization
14. registered dietitian
15. federal health insurance for persons with low incomes
17. short procedure unit
18. number of years education required for PT, OT and speech therapy
20. respiratory therapist
24. common illness requiring rehabilitation
25. occupational therapist
27. electrocardiogram
28. radiograph

Health-Care System: Short Answer

Answer the following questions in the space provided.

20. Fragmentation of care can be confusing, disruptive and potentially dangerous to the client. Identify how a nurse might intervene to reduce the number of problems resulting from fragmentation of care.

21. Explain why private health insurance is referred to as ***third-party reimbursement.***

22. Under what conditions is referral to hospice care appropriate?

23. List the three levels of care which are the primary focus of long-term care centers.
    a.
    b.
    c.

24. Differentiate between Government financing for health care in Canada and the United States.

Canadian Health Care Financing	US Health Care Financing

Health-Care Agency: Sentence Completion

Complete the sentences below by providing the appropriate word or phrase.

25. In ____ (year) Medicare converted to a prospective payment plan, referred to as __________ __________ __________.

26. The Multiple Sclerosis Society, International Red Cross, Canadian Lung Association, Cystic Fibrosis Society are all nonprofit organizations referred to as __________ _____ agencies.

Health-Care Team

Complete the table below by supplying the missing information.

Health Team Member	Role	Education	License /Title
27. Pharmacist	a.	b.	c.
28. Physical Therapist	a.	b.	c.
29. Physicians' Assistant	a.	b.	c.
30. Occupational Therapist	a.	b.	c.
31. Dietitian	a.	b.	c.
32. Respiratory Therapist	a.	b.	c.

Additional Enrichment Activities

1. Assemble a list of mutual self-help group meeting times from local/community centers. Select one to attend. Share your observations with your classmates.
2. Select one long-term care facility or adult day-care center in your area. Determine who makes up the health-care team in that particular facility.
3. Locate a pamphlet on Medicare reimbursements. Become familiar with it and file for future reference.
4. Update your classmates on the role/education/accountability of the new health care worker called the "Registered Clinical Technician" (RCT) proposed by the American Medical Association in 1988. What is the American Nurses' Association's response to this new category of worker?

Suggested Readings

Alleyne GAO: Health problems old and new. World Health October: 9-10, 1987

Brider P: Too poor to pay: The scandal of patient dumping. AJN 87(11):1147-51, 1987

Califano JA: Health care revolution: Nursing & Health Care 8(7):400-06, 1987

Cary AH: Preparation for professional practice: what do we need? Nursing Clinics of North America 23(3):391-51, 1988

Joel LA: Reshaping nursing practice. AJN 87(6):793-795, 1987

Phillips EK et al: DRG ripple effects on community health nursing. Public Health Nursing 4(2):4-8, 1987

Roper WL: Medicare tomorrow. Nursing & Health Care 8(7):412-14, 1987

Spitzer R: Nursing productivity : The hospital's key to survival and profit. Chicago, S-N Publications, 1986

Warner SL: Third party payments: untangling the web. Nursing & Health Care 9:(4)180-84, 1988

Williamson GC et al: Health care cost containment: Current societal forces and health care trends. AAOHN Journal 35(10):444-8, 1987

Chapter 4
Theoretical Base for Nursing Practice

Chapter 4 of Fundamentals of Nursing (Taylor, 1988) explores the unique *knowledge base* of nursing that provides the rationales for nursing activities. Nursing theories are introduced as the organizing framework for the practice of nursing.
After studying this chapter and completing the workbook exercises, the learner should be able to

- Define key terms used in the chapter.
- Describe the underlying processes and characteristics of nursing theory.
- Define the four common components of nursing theory.
- Summarize the historical background, cultural influences, and value of nursing theory.
- Discuss selected nursing theories, including definitions, assumptions, beliefs, and applications to nursing practice.

Key Terms Chapter 4

adaptation theory
concept
conceptual framework or model
developmental theory
environment
general systems theory
health
nursing
nursing theory
person
philosophy
process
theory

Nursing Theory: Match

Match the terms with the appropriate definitions.

a. adaptation theory
b. concepts
c. conceptual framework
d. developmental theory
e. environment
f. general systems theory
g. nursing
h. nursing theory
i. person
j. philosophy
k. process
l. theory
m. autonomous
n. deductive reasoning

1. ____ Attempts to describe or explain nursing.
2. ____ Explains the breaking of whole things into parts and then learning how the parts work together.
3. ____ According to Roy, a biophysical being and an integrated whole.
4. ____ Ideas.
5. ____ According to Orem, modern society's values and expectations.
6. ____ A dynamic or continuously changing process that effects change and involves interactions and response.
7. ____ A group of concepts that follows an understandable pattern.
8. ____ A group of concepts that form a pattern of reality.
9. ____ Being independent and self-governing.
10. ____ The study of wisdom, fundamental knowledge, and the processes used to develop and construct our perceptions of life.
11. ____ A method of theory development in which an idea is examined after ideas are considered.
12. ____ The actions phase of a conceptual framework.
13. ____ States that the growth and development of humans is orderly and predictable.
14. ____ A unique health-care discipline in which a service, based on knowledge and skill, is provided to others.

Nursing Theory: Completion

Answer the following questions in the space provided.

15. List the four common components of all nursing theories that influence and determine nursing practice. Circle the component that is the most significant.

a. ______________________________
b. ______________________________
c. ______________________________
d. ______________________________

16. Name three major trends that provided the impetus for the development of nursing theory.
    a. ____
    ____
    b. ____
    ____
    c. ____
    ____
17. What was the name of the first nursing research journal?
    ____
    In what year was the first nursing research journal published? __________
18. Human adaptation occurs on what three levels?
    a. ____
    b. ____
    c. ____
19. Name the five basic characteristics of nursing theory.
    a. ____
    b. ____
    c. ____
    d. ____
    e. ____

Theoretical Model: True/False

In the space provided indicate whether each statement below is TRUE or FALSE.

20. _____ The Betty Neuman model is an example of a closed system.
21. _____ Developmental theory begins with birth and ends with death.
22. _____ Maslow's theory of human needs is divided by chronological age.
23. _____ Systems are hierarchical in nature.
24. _____ Erik Erikson based his theory of psychosocial development on the process of socialization.
25. _____ If theory-based nursing is practiced, nurses work toward individual goals.

Additional Enrichment Activities

1. Determine the theoretical framework for nursing at your school and at your clinical institution. How do they differ?

2. Ask two different nurses in your clinical institution what the institution's conceptual framework for nursing is. Did they know? Why do you think this is an important issue?
3. Write your own philosophy of nursing.

Suggested Readings

Benner P, Tanner C: Clinical judgment: How expert nurses use intuition. AJN 87(1):23-31, 1987

Chinn PL et al: Theory and Nursing, St. Louis, C.V. Mosby, 1987

Fitzpatrick J and Whall A: Conceptual models of nursing: Analysis and application. Bowie, Maryland, Robert J. Brady Co. 1983

Krieger D: Foundations for holistic health nursing practice, Philadelphia, JB Lippincott Company, 1981

Newman B: The Newman systems model: Application to nursing education and practice. Norwalk, Connecticut, Appleton-Century-Crofts, 1982

Orem D: Nursing: Concepts and practices, 2nd ed. New York, McGraw-Hill Book Company, 1980

Randell B et al: Adaptation nursing: the Roy conceptual model applied. St. Louis, C.V.Mosby Company, 1982

Roy SC, Roberts S: Theory construction in nursing, Englewood Cliffs, New Jersey, Prentice Hall, Inc., 1981

Steiger NJ, Lipson JG: Self-care nursing theory and practice. Bowie, Maryland, Brady Communications Company, Inc., 1985

Stevens BJ: Nursing theory 2nd ed Boston, Little, Brown and Company, 1984

Computer Assisted Instructions

Fundamentals of Nursing Theory. Upgrade Unlimited, Inc.

Chapter 5
Values and Ethics in Nursing

In chapter 5 of Fundamentals of Nursing (Taylor 1988), the learner is exposed to the ethical dimensions of nursing practice. Because nursing activities place the nurse in situations that demand sensitivity to the value-laden health care decision making process, the impact of values on human behavior is a significant factor in nursing practice.

After studying this chapter and completing the workbook exercises, the learner will be able to

- Define key terms used in the chapter.
- Explain how the six basic value orientations can result in persons in the same situation responding differently.
- Identify five common modes of value transmission.
- Describe the seven steps in the valuing process.
- Identify the seven basic values essential in the practice of nursing.
- Utilize values clarification strategies in clinical practice.
- Describe professional ethical conduct.
- Describe how different sources of moral authority may reach different decisions regarding ethical problems.
- Recognize ethical issues as they arise in nursing practice.
- Utilize a nursing code of ethics to guide nursing actions.
- Utilize an ethical framework/model to assist in the assessment and resolution of ethical dilemmas.
- Respect valid alternatives for solving the ethical problems that arise in clinical practice.

Key Terms Chapter 5

You will become familiar with the meaning of the following terms used in this chapter.

advocacy
attitude
autonomy
beliefs
beneficence
confidentiality
ethics
fidelity
justice
morals
nonmaleficence
utilitarianism
value
value system
values clarification
veracity

Values and Ethics : Matching

Match the terms with the appropriate definition.

Terms:

a. advocacy
b. attitude
c. autonomy
d. beliefs
e. beneficence
f. confidentiality
g. ethics
h. morals
i. nonmaleficence
j. utilitarianism
k. value
l. value system
m. values clarification
n. veracity

Definitions:

1. ____ truth telling
2. ____ a process by which persons come to understand their own values and value system
3. ____ a special class of intellectual attitudes based primarily on faith as opposed to fact
4. ____ respecting privileged information
5. ____ the greatest good for the greatest number
6. ____ the protection and support of another's rights
7. ____ a feeling or an emotion
8. ____ personal standards
9. ____ self-determination
10. ____ doing good
11. ____ a personal belief about worth that acts as a standard to guide one's behavior
12. ____ avoiding harm
13. ____ a system dealing with professional standards of behavior related to what is right and wrong
14. ____ an organization of values in which each value is ranked along a continuum of importance

Values and Ethics: True/False

Indicate whether the statement is TRUE or FALSE.

15. _____ Ethics provide clear-cut answers for resolving ethical problems.
16. _____ The more complex the dilemma, the more likely it is that several courses of action can be justified as being morally right.
17. _____ We are all born with our values.
18. _____ The Patient's Bill of Rights guarantees for the patient the treatment he has a right to expect.
19. _____ Moral distress is where the nurse is unsure of which moral principles apply.
20. _____ Conventional principles do not apply to nursing.
21. _____ Distributive justice is the type of justice most relevant to health care.

Values Clarification and Ethics in Nursing : Completion

Answer the following questions in the space provided.

22. Name the six value orientations described in your text.
    a. ______________________________
    b. ______________________________
    c. ______________________________
    d. ______________________________
    e. ______________________________
    f. ______________________________
23. Name the five common modes of value transmission.
    a. ______________________________
    b. ______________________________
    c. ______________________________
    d. ______________________________
    e. ______________________________
24. Identify the three main activities on which the process of valuing is focused.
    a. ______________________________
    b. ______________________________
    c. ______________________________
25. Describe the seven steps of the valuing process.
    a. ______________________________
    b. ______________________________
    c. ______________________________
    d. ______________________________

e. ____________________

f. ____________________

g. ____________________

26. List seven basic values essential in the practice of nursing.

a. ____________________

b. ____________________

c. ____________________

d. ____________________

e. ____________________

f. ____________________

g. ____________________

27. Explain what is meant by professional ethical conduct.

28. Why do you think the President's Commission for the Study of Ethical Problems rejects placing absolute authority for decisions in the hands of the client?

Case Study

Mrs. Holmes, a 70 year-old widow, was diagnosed with advanced cancer of the esophagus. She is scheduled for surgery which she knows is not curative, but may prolong her life.

Prior to surgery, Mrs. Holmes becomes withdrawn and tearful. She tells you she is not sure she wants to go through with surgery. She shares with you that she's had a long and happy life, and can accept her death. She asks you to help her decide what to do.
You believe you must do everything possible to help Mrs. Holmes, but you know that she has the right to make her own decisions.

For each intervention given in the table below check either *Yes* if you believe it should be implemented, or *No* of you believe the interventions suggested should NOT be implemented. Provide the rationale for your decision in the last column of the table.

Nursing Interventions	Yes	No	Rationale
29. Ask for your assignment to be changed.			
30. Help Mrs. Holmes problem solve, assess her fears and understanding of the implications of having or not having surgery.			
31. Tell Mrs. Holmes she should have the surgery.			
32. Support Mrs. Holmes in whatever decision she makes.			
33. Talk to Mrs. Holmes' family, ask them to convince her to have the surgery.			
34. Suggest a conference to include Mrs. Holmes, her family, her physician, and yourself to discuss surgery.			
35. Acknowledge her right to decide as well as the right to change her mind. Assure her that care will be available in either event.			
36. Tell her she will get better after the surgery and to stop worrying.			

Additional Enrichment Activities

1. Complete the questions on page 104 of Fundamentals of Nursing (Taylor, 1988) regarding values guiding your professional behavior. Compare these to the philosophy you wrote for a previous assignment.
2. If there is an ethics committee at your institution, find out what type of professionals serve on it. Is nursing represented? What is the procedure for seeking their assistance?
3. Identify a moral dilemma which you are currently experiencing. Utilize Jameton's model in reaching a decision about your dilemma.

Suggested Readings

American Nurses' Association, Dilemmas in practice: Withdrawing or withholding food and fluid. AJN 88(6):797-804, 1988

Anderson RC et al: Ethical issues in health promotion and health education. AAOHN J 35(5):220-31, 246-8, 1987

Clough JG: Making life and death decisions you can live with. RN 51(5):28-30, 1988

Erikson I, Mitchell C: Dilemmas in practice: Which child gets the transplant? AJN 88:88(3):287-95, 1988

Hard choices: ethical issues in nutritional support (Case study) Nutrition Supp Serv 7(2):19-21, 1987

Smurl JF: Making hard choices, finding solutions to every day ethical problems, Nursing 18(6):105-8, 1988

Steele SM: Clarifying values. Nursing & Health Care 7(5):246-249, 1986

Chapter 6
Legal Implications of Nursing

The legal accountability of nurses is the focus of Chapter 6 of Fundamentals of Nursing (Taylor, 1988).

After studying this chapter and completing the workbook exercises, the learner should be able to

- Define key terms used in the chapter.
- Define law, describing its four sources.
- Describe the professional and legal regulation of nursing practice.
- Identify the purpose of credentialing; using as examples accreditation, licensure/registration, and certification.
- Identify grounds for suspending or revoking a license or registration.
- Differentiate intentional torts (assault and battery, defamation, invasion of privacy, false imprisonment, fraud) and unintentional torts (negligence).
- Evaluate personal areas of potential liability in nursing.
- Describe the legal procedure once a plaintiff files a complaint against a nurse for negligence.
- Describe the roles of the nurse as defendant, fact witness, and expert witness.
- Understand the need for use of appropriate legal safeguards in nursing practice (competent practice within scope defined by nurse practice act, careful documentation, participation in risk management programs, use of professional liability insurance).
- Explain the purpose of incident reports.
- Describe laws affecting nursing practice.

Key Terms Chapter 6

assault
battery
civil law
common law
credentialing
crime
defamation of character
defendant
false imprisonment
felony
fraud
incident reports
informed consent
invasion of privacy
law
liability
licensure
litigation
living will
malpractice
misdemeanor
negligence
plaintiff
public law
risk management
standard of care
statutory law
tort

Legal Implications of Nursing: Match

Match the terms with the appropriate definitions.

Terms:

a. assault
b. battery
c. civil law
d. common law
e. credentialing
f. crime
g. defamation of character
h. defendant
i. false imprisonment
j. felony
k. fraud
l. incident report
m. informed consent
n. invasion of privacy
o. law
p. liability
q. licensure
r. litigation
s. living will
t. malpractice
u. misdemeanor
v. negligence
w. plaintiff
x. public law
y. risk management

Definitions:

1. ____ a general term that refers to ways in which professional competence is ensured and maintained
2. ____ a wrong against a person or his property
3. ____ unintentional torts
4. ____ a threat or an attempt to make bodily contact with another person without that person's consent
5. ____ willful and purposeful misrepresentation that could cause, or has caused, loss or harm to a person or property
6. ____ what a reasonably prudent person would or would not have done under similar circumstances

7.____ a tool used by health-care institutions to document the occurrence of anything "out of the ordinary" that results in or has the potential to result in harm
8. ____ a law in which the government is directly involved
9. ____ the person or government bringing suit against another
10. ____ the process of a lawsuit
11. ____ court-made law
12. ____ the one being accused of a crime or tort
13. ____ the process by which a state determines that a candidate meets certain minimum requirements to practice in the profession of his or her choice and grants a license to do so
14. ____ a crime less serious than a felony
15. ____ a standard or rule of conduct established and enforced by the government or a society
16. ____ a crime punishable by imprisonment in a state or federal penitentiary for more than one year
17. ____ an assault that is carried out and includes every willful, angry, and violent or negligent touching of other's person or clothes or anything attached to or held by that person
18. ____ an intentional tort in which one party makes derogatory remarks about another, diminishing the other party's reputation
19. ____ involves disclosure, comprehension, competence, and voluntary action
20. ____ disclosure of confidential information whenever a client's problem is inappropriately discussed with a third party
21. ____ consists of duty, breach of duty, causation, and damages
22. ____ consists of safety program, products safety program, and quality assurance program
23. ____ describes a person's wishes with regard to being kept alive by artificial means or heroic measures when there is no reasonable expectation of recovery from a physical or mental disability
24. ____ private law that regulates the relationships among people
25. ____ unjustified retention or prevention of the movement of another person without proper consent
26. ____ negligence of professional personnel

Legal Aspects of Nursing: True/False

Indicate whether the statement below is TRUE or FALSE.

27. ____ A tort is a wrong committed against another person.
28. ____ Statutory laws are enacted by legislative bodies.
29. ____ Legislation sets requirements for licensure/registration of nurses.
30. ____ Invasion of privacy is an unintentional tort.
31. ____ A patient is adequately informed after the consent form is signed.

32. ____ Documentation of the consent process through the use of a printed consent form constitutes informed consent.
33. ____ Breach of duty is the failure to meet the standards of care.
34. ____ A student nurse is held to the same standard of care as the registered nurse.

Short Answer Questions

Answer the following questions in the space provided.

35. Name the four sources of law.
    a. ______
    b. ______
    c. ______
    d. ______
36. List the reasons the State Board of Nurse Examiners may revoke or suspend a nurse's license.

    ______
37. When is a signed consent form needed in a hospital? Why can't one form cover every thing?

    ______
38. List the four necessary elements of informed consent.
    a. ______
    b. ______
    c. ______
    d. ______
39. Liability consists of four elements. Name them.
    a. ______

b. __________
c. __________
d. __________

40. What are some recommendations for the nurse defendant in a legal case?

41. Discuss the meaning of risk management.

42. What are the elements of a comprehensive risk management program?

43. List eight elements of competent practice.
a. __________
b. __________
c. __________
d. __________
e. __________
f. __________
g. __________
h. __________

Additional Enrichment Activities

1. Obtain an admission consent form from your clinical facility. How is it different from a special procedure consent form?
2. To comply with quality assurance at your institution, there are certain items that must be documented on each patient every shift. Find out what these are.
3. Obtain a copy of a living will form. Become familiar enough with it to answer clients questions.
4. Check your institutional policy for restraining a patient.
5. Observe the news media (newspapers, periodicals, television and radio) for items pertaining to malpractice, liability suits, and other legal action involving health care personnel and institutions. Bring clippings, reviews to class for discussion and bulletin board display.

Suggested Readings

Bennett HM: The legal liabilities of the Good Samaritan Act. Home Healthcare Nurse 1(1):47, 1983

Cushing M: The legal side: Short-staffing on trial. AJN 88(2):161-69, 1988

Cushing M: The legal side: Nurses have rights, too. AJN 88(2):167-75, 1988

Dean KA: Informed consent. Focus on Critical Care 10(4):62-63, 1983

Goldstein A, Pruitt S: Nurses legal advisor. Philadelphia, JB Lippincott Company, 1988

Creighton H: Legal significance of charging. Nursing Management 18(9):17, 20, 22, 1987

Northrop, CE: Did negligence cause the patient's fall? Nursing '87 17(11):43, 1987

Northrop CE, Kelly ME: Legal issues in nursing. AJN 87(12):1583, 1987

Varga K: How to protect yourself against malpractice.....students of nursing. Imprint 31(2):84-88, 1984

Unit II
The Client: Concepts for Holistic Care

Unit II focuses on the consumer of health care, the client. Concepts basic to providing holistic care for the client, i.e., basic human needs, culture and ethnicity, stress and adaptation, are considered in Chapter 7, 8, and 9 respectively.

Chapter 7
Human Needs:
Person, Family, and Community

After studying this chapter in Fundamentals of Nursing (Taylor, 1988) and completing the associated workbook exercises the student should be able to

- Define key terms used in the chapter.
- Describe each level of Maslow's hierarchy of basic human needs.
- Discuss nursing actions necessary to meet needs for each level of the hierarchy.
- Define family concepts, including family role, structures, functions, developmental stages/tasks, and risk factors.
- Identify aspects of the community that impact individual and family health.
- Describe nursing interventions to promote and maintain health in the individual, the family, and the community.

Key Terms Chapter 7

basic human needs
blended family
cohabiting family
community
extended family
human sexuality
love and belonging needs
nuclear family
physiologic needs
safety and security needs
self-actualization needs
single-parent family
traditional family

Chapter 7 Key Terms Crossword Puzzle

Complete the crossword puzzle, using Key Terms from Chapter 7.

Across

1. A physiologic need that is a component of health is human _____ .
3. Living together
6. The need to feel good about oneself is self-_____.
7. Divorced individuals marry with each bringing children into the new family. The new family structure is referred to as a _____ family.
8. _____ _____ _____ are those needs common to all people, prioritized by Maslow from highest to lowest.
11. The _____ family, a father, mother and children, married and living in one household represents 73% of all households.
12. The most basic of all are the _____ needs.
14. The nuclear and extended families are examples of a _____ family structure.

Down

2. The _____ family includes aunts, uncles, cousins and other relatives who may or may not live with the nuclear family.
3. A person, as an individual and as a member of a family, belongs to a _____.
4. The next highest need after safety and security is the need for love and _____.
5. A "hierarchy of _____" suggests that some _____ are more important than others.
9. Self-_____ is the need to reach one's potential through developing one's unique capabilities.
10. Removing environmental hazards, such as spills, meets a clients _____ and security needs.
13. One example of an alternate family structure is the _____ parent family.

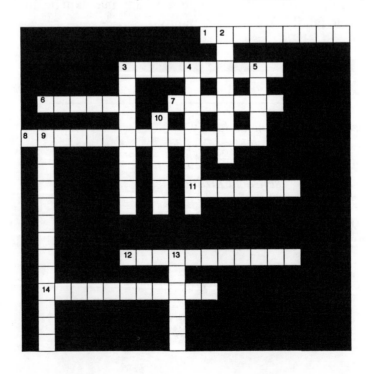

Family Functions Table

Complete the table below by providing an example of how the *family functions* could be met in a family.

Family Functions	Examples
14. Physical	______________
15. Economic	______________
16. Reproductive	______________
17. Affective/coping	______________
18. Socialization	______________

Family Risk Factors

Family risk factors are categorized into one of four categories, life-style, biologic, environmental, or social/psychological factors. Identify the correct category for each of the family risk factors in the list below by placing the corresponding first letter of the category (L, P, E, or B) in the space provided in front of the family risk factor.

Family Risk Factors

19. ____ Birth defects
20. ____ Chemical dependence
21. ____ Inadequate child-care resources
22. ____ Crowded living conditions
23. ____ Conflict between family members
24. ____ Lack of knowledge about sexual roles
25. ____ Inadequate nutrition, "junkfood" diet
26. ____ Mental retardation
27. ____ Genetic predisposition to sickle cell anemia
28. ____ Child abuse
29. ____ Water pollution

Risk Factor Categories
Life-style (**L**)
Social/Psychological (**S**)
Environmental (**E**)
Biologic (**B**)

Additional Enrichment Activities

1. In the clinical agency to which you are assigned, observe the nurses and examine the care plans to see how the family's needs are considered. How is the family included in meeting the client's needs?

2. Look in the telephone book under government agencies. Make a list of the agencies or departments in your community that are responsible for maintaining a healthy environment.
3. Interview a home health nurse, a school nurse, an industrial nurse. Ask (a) What are your clients like? (b) What is a typical day for you? (c) What do you like most/least about your job? Compare your interviews with those of your classmates who have interviewed different nurses.

Suggested Readings

Bowdler JE et al: Health needs of homeless persons. Public Health Nursing 4(3):135-40, 1987

Fagin CM: Stress: Implications for nursing research. Image 19(1):38-41, 1987

Fletcher J: Stress management. Intensive Care Nursing 3(2):56-60, 1987

Graffman S et al: A comparison of two relaxation strategies for relief of pain and its distress. J of Pain and Symptom Management 2(4):299-31, 1987.

Grey M, Hayman LL: Assessing stress in children: Research and clinical implications. J of Pediatric Nursing 2(5):316-327, 1987

Larkin J: Factors influencing one's ability to adapt to chronic illness. Nursing Clinics of North America 22(3):535-42, 1987

Pollock SE: Human responses to chronic illness: physiologic and psychosocial adaptation. Nursing Research 35(2):90-97, 1986

Swinford P: Relaxation and positive imagery for the surgical patient: a research study. Perioperative Nursing Quarterly 3(3):9-16, 1987

White DM: Health promotion pays: 3 to 1 return seen in stress management programs. Occupational Health SAF 55(8):18-9, 1986

Chapter 8
Culture and Ethnicity

The concepts presented in this chapter of the Fundamentals of Nursing (Taylor, 1988) text expose the learner to the cross-cultural aspects of nursing in a multi-cultural environment. After studying this chapter in Fundamentals of Nursing and completing the workbook exercises the learner should be able to

- Define key terms used in the chapter.
- Describe the concepts of stereotyping and ethnocentrism.
- Identify cultural norms of the health-care system.
- Discuss the importance of culture in holistic nursing care, incorporating socioeconomic, psychosocial, and ethnic/racial factors.
- Define the "culture of poverty" as it specifically relates to the issues of power and health care.
- List physiologic and psychosocial health risks common to certain ethnic/racial populations.
- Discuss the significance of cultural health beliefs and traditional folk medicine for clients entering the health-care system.
- Describe key concepts and specific guidelines for giving transcultural nursing care.

Key Terms Chapter 8

You will want to become familiar with the meaning of the following key terms used in this chapter.

culture	*holism*	*stereotyping*
culture shock	*holistic health care*	*subculture*
ethnic group	*humanism*	*Yin and Yang*
ethnocentrism	*race*	

Definitions of Key Terms

Define the following terms.

1. Humanism

___

2. Race

___

3. Ethnic Group

___

4. Culture

___

5. Subculture

___

6. Stereotyping

___

7. Ethnocentrism

___

Classification of Cultural Terms

Place the terms listed below in the appropriate category in the table.

8. white
9. Irish
10. black
11. drug users
12. rural black
13. street people
14. Jewish
15. urban poor
16. yellow
17. bag ladies
18. Mexican-Americans

CATEGORY

Race	Ethnic Group	Culture	Subculture

Poverty defined

19. Define poverty on the basis of income.

____

____

____

20. Define poverty on the basis of attitudes of individuals and communities.

____

____

____

21. Describe poverty as a power issue.

____

____

____

22. List three groups in America who are especially likely to be poor. Discuss the reasons for their poverty.

Group **Reasons for Poverty**

a. ____

b. ____

c. ____

Race/Ethnic Group Match

Match the disease/condition with the race or ethnic group it is most likely to affect. There may be more than one group for each disease.

23. Tay-Sachs Disease ____
24. Sickle Cell Anemia ____
25. Lactase Deficiency ____
26. Gout
27. G-6-PD Deficiency ____
28. Thalassemia ____
29. Sarcoidosis ____
30. Keloid Formation ____

A.	**Afro-American**
B.	**Eastern European Jews**
C.	**White Female**
D.	**Asians**
E.	**White Males**
F.	**Mediterranean**
G.	**Puerto Rican Males**
H	**Filipino Males**

Implementing cross-cultural considerations

31. Discuss several ways in which the nurse could incorporate cross-cultural considerations into the care plan for a client.

____

____

____

____

____

____

Additional Enrichment Activities

1. In the agency you are assigned to for clinical, examine the nursing assessment forms (admission data bases) to see how much cultural information they will elicit. List the specific areas of the forms that elicit this data. Do the same for the nursing assessment forms used by your nursing school. Would a "cultural assessment tool" be needed, or do these forms provide enough data?
2. During one clinical day, list all the examples of stereotyping or ethnocentrism you see.
3. Describe some examples of folk medicine used by your family and friends.
4. Make a list of the ethnic groups and subcultures you can identify in your community.

Suggested Readings

Anthony-Tkach C: Nursing and health care in the Soviet Union. Nursing Forum 22(2):45-52, 1985

Fowler MDV, Levine-Ariff J: Ethics at the bedside: A source book for the critical care nurse. Philadelphia, JB Lippincott Company987

Holtzen VL: A comparative study of nursing in China and the United States. Nursing Forum 22(3):86-93, 1985

Popp R: Health care for the poor: where has all the money gone? J Nursing Administration 18(1):8-12, 1988

Tien-Hyatt J: Keying in on the unique care needs of Asian clients. Nursing and Health Care 8(5):268-71, 1987

Chapter 9
Stress and Adaptation

Health care settings are filled with clients who are experiencing a variety of forms of stress and it is important for nurses to have knowledge of the dimensions of stress and how stress impacts on individuals. After studying this chapter of Fundamentals of Nursing (Taylor, 1988) and completing the workbook exercises the learner should be able to

- Define key terms used in the chapter.
- Describe the mechanisms involved in maintaining physiologic homeostasis.
- Explain the interdependent nature of stressors, stress, and adaptation.
- Compare and contrast developmental and situational stress, incorporating the concepts of physiologic and psychosocial stressors.
- Describe the physical and emotional responses to stress, including mind-body interaction, local adaptation syndrome, general adaptation syndrome, and coping/defense mechanisms.
- Discuss the effects of short- and long-term stress on basic human needs, health and illness, and the family.
- Integrate knowledge of healthy life-style, support systems, stress management techniques, and crisis intervention into nursing care plans.
- Recognize and effectively cope with stress unique to the nursing profession.

Key Terms Chapter 9

adaptation
anxiety
burnout
coping mechanisms
crisis
crisis intervention
defense mechanisms
developmental crisis
"fight or flight" response
general adaptation syndrome (GAS)
homeostasis
inflammatory response
local adaptation syndrome (LAS)
psychosomatic disorders
reflex pain response
situational stress
stress
stressor

Key Terms Scramblegram

Find the words that fit the blanks. They may appear diagonally, horizontally, vertically, backwards, etc. A sample puzzle is shown at the right.

Sample:
1. A term used in football is (offside).

O	A	B	T
F	C	L	D
F	A	E	F
S	I	D	E

1. ____________ is the series of responses a person makes to maintain balance when there is stress.
2. ____________is a vague sense of impending doom.
3. Nurses who are overwhelmed by on-the-job stressors may develop ____________ .
4. Smoking, crying, and laughing are examples of ____________ used to handle mild anxiety.
5. When the usual coping and defense mechanisms fail, a ____________ occurs.
6. Crisis ____________________ is a 5-step problem-solving technique.
7. ____________ are used in mild to moderate anxiety to protect the self. Used to extreme, they may become maladaptive.
8. ____________crises occur as a person progresses through the normal stages from birth to old age.
9. When the body prepares to resist or run away in the face of a stressor, this is called the "________________ " response.
10. Hans Selye developed the model of stress called the General ________________ Syndrome. (abbreviation)
11. ________________ is the essential balance in the internal environment of the body, needed to maintain life.
12. One example of the LAS is the ______________________ response. Another is the ______________ pain response.
13. The __________________ adaptation syndrome (or _ _ _) involves a body part, (tissue / organ), not the whole body.

14. Chronic diarrhea and asthma are examples of ______________ disorders, partly due to psychological influences.
15. ______________ is a condition in which the person responds to changes in his/her normal balanced state.
16. A _____ is anything that causes a person to experience a change in his/her balanced state.

```
RFIGHTORFLIGHTAS
BENCDISORDERSDMI
EFFGHIJSKLMNOSPS
NQLLRSTSUVWXIIYI
OZAOEABECDLNENFR
IGMHCXIRJKALMTNC
TOMPQARTSHSTRESS
ATAUVWLSCXYZARBC
TDTLATNEMPOLEVED
PEOFGHMIJKLMNEOE
APRQRGASSTUVWNXF
DYYZNABBURNOUTCE
ANXIETYDEFGHIIJN
KLPMNADAPTATIONS
HOMEOSTASISOPNQE
CRSTUVSMSINAHCEM
```

Defense Mechanism Match

Match the defense mechanisms to the example behaviors.

Defense Mechanisms

A. Compensation
B. Displacement
C. Denial
D. Introjection
E. Projection
F. Regression
G. Reaction formation
H. Rationalization
I. Suppression

Example Behaviors:

17. ____ A man with a heart attack keeps insisting, "It's only indigestion."
18. ____ "There's no money to pay the bills, but I'll think about it tomorrow."
19. ____ A nursing student is disappointed with her test grade. She stomps her foot, cries, and does not look at the instructor all during class.
20. ____ Disappointed that she has lost no weight after trying a low-calorie diet for two weeks the client says, "Oh well, my husband likes me this size anyway."
21. ____ Disappointed with a 75% test grade, a student says, "The instructor doesn't like me or she wouldn't have graded me so hard."

22. _____ The student receives her grades in the mail. They are not good. She kicks the dog.

Stress Short Answer

Explain how the following activities can be used to reduce stress.

23. Exercise ______________________________
24. Rest and sleep ______________________________
25. Nutrition ______________________________

Crisis Intervention

List the 5 steps of crisis intervention.

26. ______________________________
27. ______________________________
28. ______________________________
29. ______________________________
30. ______________________________

Physiologic Effects of Stress

Match the body system/organ with its effect on the body during stress.

A. Sympathetic nervous system
B. Pituitary Gland
C. Adrenal Medulla
D. Adrenal Cortex

31. ____ Stimulates the adrenal cortex
32. ____ Dilates blood vessels in skeletal muscle
33. ____ Produces glucocorticoid to raise glucose levels for energy
34. ____ Produces epinephrine to support the sympathetic nervous system
35. ____ Produces aldosterone to regulate fluid and electrolytes

Additional Enrichment Activities

1. Look in the telephone book to see which of the support groups on page 233 of your text can be found in your community. Arrange to attend a meeting or talk with someone who works there, if possible. If this is not possible, obtain literature about the group. Find out what kind of crises the group deals with and how they provide support to those in crisis.
2. Make a list of the coping mechanisms you use when you are:
   a. Mildly anxious
   b. Very anxious
   Compare these with behaviors you see in your assigned clients.
3. In clinical, identify a patient who is anxious, in pain, restless, or unable to fall asleep. Teach the patient to use the deep breathing and/or progressive muscle relaxation techniques on page 233 of your text. Report in post conference, the patient's response to these techniques.

Suggested Readings

Fagin CM: Stress: Implications for nursing research. Image 19(1):38-41, 1987

Fletcher J: Stress management. Intensive Care Nursing 3(2):56-60, 1987

Grey M, Hayman L: Assessing stress in children: Research and clinical applications. J of Pediatric Nursing 2(5):316-27, 1987

McCranie E et al: Work stress, hardiness, and burnout among hospital staff nurses. Nursing Research 36(6):374-379, 1987

Pollock SE: Human responses to chronic illness: Physiologic and psychosocial adaptation. Nursing Research 35(2):90-97, 1987

White DM: Health promotion pays: 3-1 return seen in stress management programs. Occupations Health SAF 55(8):18-9, 1986

Unit III
Promoting Wellness Across the Lifespan

Nurses give care to clients and their families at all ages and stages of growth and development throughout the lifespan, during health and wellness. Developmental theories provide the guidelines for giving individualized nursing care taking into consideration the family constellation and relationships, as well as the physiologic, cognitive, psychosocial, moral, and spiritual components of the individual. The four chapters in this unit take the learner sequentially through the stages of growth and development. Recognizing the increasing number of persons over the age of 65, Chapter 12 focuses upon the developmental stages of older adults and associated nursing interventions. Chapter 13 deals with death as the final stage of life.

Chapter 10
Developmental Concepts

Nurses care for persons of all ages and stages of development whether as individuals or as families. Regardless, each individual brings a unique set of concerns, needs, hopes and fears to the nurse-client relationship. In this chapter of Fundamentals of Nursing (Taylor, 1988) the learner is introduced to basic principles of growth and development, which serve as the foundation for understanding human behavior.

After studying this chapter and completing the workbook exercises the learner should be able to

- Define key terms used in the chapter.
- Summarize basic principles of growth and development.
- Discuss the theories of Freud, Piaget, Havighurst, Erikson, Kohlberg, and Fowler.
- Describe the importance of incorporating multiple theories of growth and development in assessing and planning nursing care for an individual client.
- Describe the dynamics of family in providing nursing care.
- List implications for nursing practice that derive from a knowledge of growth and development.

Key Terms Chapter 10

You will want to become familiar with the meaning of the following key terms used in this chapter.

accommodation	*growth*
assimilation	*maturation*
cognitive development	*moral development*
developmental task	*psychosocial theory*
faith	*sexuality*

Developmental Theories: Matching

Match the behavior with the developmental theory/principle in the following matching sections/

Developmental Theories: Erikson, Freud, Havighurst

Developmental Theory/Principle

a. Erikson's Ego Integrity vs Despair
b. Development is cephalocaudal in direction
c. Erikson's Autonomy vs. Shame and Doubt
d. Freud's Phallic stage
e. Freud's Latency stage
f. Freud's Id
g. There are periods of growth and development vulnerable to certain stimuli
h. Growth and development is orderly and sequential
i. Erikson's Industry vs. Inferiority

Behavior

1. ____ a child mimics sounds before he speaks words
2. ____ a newborn bonds with his mother during the first hour of life
3. ____ an elderly person reviews his life events and decides it was all worthwhile
4. ____ a nine year old plays Monopoly with his peers
5. ____ a 15 month old infant is learning to walk
6. ____ a two year old's favorite word is "No"
7. ____ an eight year old girls identifies with her mother
8. ____ a newborn cries with hunger
9. ____ a five year old masturbates
10. ____ an infant achieves head control before control of his hands and feet

Developmental Theories: Fowler, Piaget, Kohlberg

Developmental Theory/Principle

a. Piaget primary circular reaction stage
b. Fowler's synthetic-conventional faith
c. Fowler's intuitive-projective faith
d. Piaget's secondary schemata stage
f. Kohlberg's conventional level
g. Kohlberg's preconventional level
h. Piaget's secondary circular reaction stage
i. Fowler's conjunctive faith
j. Kohlberg's postconventional level

Behavior

11. ____ an adult integrates other viewpoints about faith into his own
12. ____ a preschooler refrains from dipping into the cookie jar because he knows he will be spanked if caught
13. ____ an adolescent stops at a red light
14. ____ an adult accepts the value system of others and takes responsibility for his own beliefs
15. ____ a 5 month old rattles a toy to enjoy the sound it makes
16. ____ an adult makes the statement "other people have rights too"
17. ____ an adolescent questions his parents' religion
18. ____ a 3 year old child folds his hands and bows his head to pray
19. ____ a 10 month old plays a game of "I drop and you fetch"
20. ____ a 2 month old baby smiles repeatedly in response to a human face

Case Study

Mrs. Alberti brings her 8 year old daughter Maria, 5 year old son Tonio, and 4 month old daughter Rosa, to the clinic for health checkups. Mr. Alberti has recently taken a job as a truck driver and has been absent from home for several weeks at a time. Maria, the 8 year old, is a friendly outgoing child who eagerly "helps" answer the nurse's questions; however, she shies away from the medicine cabinet, telling her brother, "the needles are kept there."

Tonio is quieter and more reserved than his sister. He shyly peeks at the nurse from behind his mother's skirts and becomes quite upset when it is his turn to be examined. Mrs. Alberti states he has been extremely possessive of her lately. He demonstrates overt resentment toward the baby and has lately asked to be held, rocked, and treated just like his baby sister.

Answer the following questions about the Alberti family in the space provided.

21. Why do you think Tonio is acting this way?

21. What stage of psychosocial development is Tonio in?

Baby Rosa is quite a "chubby" baby. Her mother proudly reports that she takes her formula very well. She is also rolling from her back to her side, grasps objects, focuses on objects, smiles and laughs, and loves the attention of her older siblings.

23. What cognitive level of development is Rosa exhibiting?

Mrs. Alberti reports that Maria is doing well in school and has many friends.

24. What stage of psychosocial development is Maria in?

25. What stage of cognitive development would apply to Maria?

26. Maria needs a booster immunization. How can the nurse best prepare her for this experience considering her present developmental stage?

Mrs. Alberti states she has noticed quite a bit of difference between Maria and Tonio in the way they perceive right and wrong.

27. What helpful information concerning the differences in the moral development levels of these two children could you provide their mother, Mrs. Alberti?

Mrs. Alberti states she tried starting Rosa on cereal per spoon last month but she didn't like it and continually spit it out.

28. What advice would you give her concerning the baby's behavior? Was she merely expressing a dislike for cereal?

Mrs. Alberti seems to demonstrate great love and concern for her family and their well-being. She is proud of their accomplishments. She also serves on school and church committees occasionally which she says allows her some socialization with women of her own age and interests.

29. In what psychosocial stage would you place Mrs. Alberti? Provide the rationale for your decision.

Mrs. Alberti states that she and her husband have recently taken in his elderly mother to live with them. She feels that it is her responsibility to help provide and care for her mother-in-law.

30. At what moral level of development would you expect Mrs. Alberti, the mother-in-law, to be functioning in?

31. What problems might you anticipate will arise in the multigenerational family?

32. In general, how will this arrangement affect the development of each family member?

Additional Enrichment Activities

1. Visit a day care center, preschool, elementary school, and high school. Observe a class of each age group. Interview some of the children individually. Look for behaviors according to the major developmental theorists discussed in this chapter of your text. Compare and contrast the different age groups.
2. Visit a meeting of a family support group of one or more of the following organizations: diabetes association, Alcoholics Anonymous, cancer society, arthritis, cystic fibrosis, asthma, heart association, etc. Identify ways family members are involved and how they are affected by the afflicted family member. Identify normal development tasks and note how these are influenced by the illness in all family members.

3. Visit a neighborhood, family, or facility of a cultural background other than your own. Interview the people you meet. Identify cultural differences that seem characteristic of the group and how they seem to impact normal developmental tasks. Assess how they might affect health and wellness.
4. Visit a retirement center. Interview some of the residents and look at their behaviors in light of the developmental theories discussed in this chapter.

Suggested Readings

Baker PD: Moral competency: an essential element in the socialization of professional nurses. Family and Community Health 10(1):8-14, 1987

Bax M: Developmental screening: baby talk. Community Outlook November:22-24, 1986

Burnard P: Encountering adults. Senior Nurse 4(4):30-31, 1988

Cherry BS, et al: Changing concepts of childhood and society. Pediatric Nursing 12(6):421-424, 1986

Gibbs NR, et al: Grays on the go. Time 12(3):44, 1988

Hindelang M: Aging: a positive experience of growth. Patient Education and Counseling, April, 9(2):209-211, 1987

Lyons JAF: Adolsecent health and school-based clinics. Issues In Comprehensive Pediatric Nursing 10(516):303-314, 1987

Nolan JW: Developmental concerns and the health of midlife women. Nursing Clinics of North America 21(1):151-159, 1986

Phillips S, et al: Developmental differences and interventions for blind children. Pediatric Nursing. May-June 14(3):201-204, 1988

Williams PD, et al: The effects of family training and support on child behavior and parent satisfaction. Archives of Psychiatric Nursing 1(2):89-97, 1987

Chapter 11
Conception to Midlife

Chapter 11 of Fundamentals of Nursing (Taylor, 1988) continues the overview and introduction to developmental theories from Chapter 10 with specific discussion relating to the various stages of growth and development from conception through midlife.
After studying this chapter and completing the workbook exercises the learner should be able to

- Define key terms used in the chapter.
- Summarize major physiologic, cognitive, psychosocial, moral and spiritual development for each age period from conception through adolescence.
- Describe the influences of play and recreation on development at specific ages.
- List common health problems of each age period through childhood requiring intervention by health practitioners.
- Identify major nursing roles specific to each period of development.
- Identify the major developmental tasks of the young and middle-adult as described by Erikson, Levinson, and Gould.
- Describe the physical, psychosocial, intellectual, moral, and spiritual development of the young adult and middle adult.
- Discuss the common health problems and nursing interventions to promote health in the adult from age 20 to 60.

Key Terms Chapter 11

You will want to become familiar with the following key terms used in this Chapter.

accommodation
acquired immune deficiency syndrome (AIDS)
active transport
andropause
anorexia nervosa
anterior fontanelle
caput succedaneum
cleft lip
cleft palate
congenital anomaly
congenital syphilis
dentition
Down's syndrome
empty-nest syndrome
failure to thrive (FTT)
fertilization
gonorrhea
herpes simplex II (genital herpes)
hypospadias
immunization
immunoglobulin
inguinal hernia
intellectualization
lanugo
linguistic
meconium
menopause
midlife crisis
milia
molding
mongolian spots
monilial infection
myelination
ossification
ovulation
physiologic jaundice
posterior fontanelle
pregnancy
prelinguistic
pseudomenstruation
puberty
quickening
reflex
school phobia
sebaceous gland
sexually transmitted disease
spermatogenesis
sphincter
spina bifida
subconjunctival hemorrhage
syphilis
temperament
trichomonal infection
trimester
vernix caseosa
visual recognition memory
widowhood

Pre-Embryonic Development

Match the germ layer in Column II with the organ it produces in Column I.

Column I
1. ___ Brain
2. ___ Intestine
3. ___ Spinal column
4. ___ Muscles
5. ___ Lungs
6. ___ Uterus
7. ___ Spinal nerves
8. ___ Bladder
9. ___ Blood vessels

Column II
A. Ectoderm
B. Mesoderm
C. Endoderm

Adult Development

Match the specific age group in Column II with the appropriate developmental phase/beliefs in Column I according to Gould's theory of adult development.

Column I
10. ___ Establishes control of self
11. ___ Demonstrates competence as an independent adult
12. ___ Questions self values (Introspective) -- time has an end
13. ___ Realization of mortality
14. ___ Increased self-confidence, no longer needs to prove self
15. ___ Set personalities special interests

Column II
A. 18-22
B. 23-28
C. 29-34
D. 35-43
E. 44-50
F. 51-60

Childhood Development: Completion

Read the questions/statements carefully and provide the best response in the space provided.

16. At what month in fetal development does each of the following developmental milestones occur?
    a. _______ Sex determination
    b. _______ Quickening
    c. _______ Fetal heart beat heard with fetoscope
    d. _______ Begins to store body fat
    e. _______ Slimmest chance of survival if born

17. The Apgar Rating Scale is routinely applied to all newborn infants at _______ minutes and _______ minutes after birth.
18. Name the five areas assessed with the Apgar Score.
    a. ____________________
    b. ____________________
    c. ____________________
    d. ____________________
    e. ____________________
19. Discuss the purpose of the Brazelton Neonatal Assessment Scale.

____
____
____
____
____
____

20. The neonatal period is defined as the time from ________to _______ .
21. Identify 4 types of health problems encountered during the neonatal period.
    a. ____________________
    b. ____________________
    c. ____________________
    d. ____________________
22. What is the purpose of the Denver Developmental Test? (DDST)

____
____
____
____
____

23. List the four areas tested by the DDST.
    a. ____________________
    b. ____________________
    c. ____________________
    d. ____________________
24. Differentiate between the terms *attachment* and *bonding*.

____
____
____
____
____

25. Discuss how differences in temperament can and do influence a child's development.

____
____
____

26. Identify the 2 most common fears experienced by hospitalized preschoolers and give examples of how the fears are manifested in behavior.
    a. __________
    b. __________

27. Describe what is meant by the term *latency child*, and identify the age group characteristic of latency.

28. How does the development of the school age child differ from most of the other developmental periods of life?

29. According to Kohlberg's theory of moral development, the school-age child starts in the ________ phase of moral development, but progresses and spends most of this period in the ________ phase of moral development.

30. What are the two focuses of orientation of the conventional phase of moral development?
    a. __________
    b. __________

31. According to Fowler, how do school-age children view religion?

32. Cite two examples of identity crisis that can occur in adolescents in our society.
    a. __________
    b. __________

33. List at least six of the developmental tasks of adolescence according to Havighurst's theory.
    a. ____________________
    b. ____________________
    c. ____________________
    d. ____________________
    e. ____________________
    f. ____________________
34. List the three leading causes of death in adolescence.
    a. ____________________
    b. ____________________
    c. ____________________
35. According to Erikson the young adult (20-30) is in the stage /crisis referred to as ________ vs ________ .
36. Five characteristics of this young adult stage of development are:
    a. ____________________
    b. ____________________
    c. ____________________
    d. ____________________
    e. ____________________
37. The middle adult (40-60) is in ______________ stage/crisis according to Erikson.
38. List at least five characteristics of the middle adult stage of development.
    a. ____________________
    b. ____________________
    c. ____________________
    d. ____________________
    e. ____________________
39. What are the two major psychosocial tasks of the young adult (20-30)?
    a. ____________________
    b. ____________________
40. The middle adult (40-60) often finds himself caught "in the middle of a generational sandwich." Discuss the significance of this phrase.

    ____
    ____
    ____
    ____
    ____
    ____

41. What are the leading causes of death in the middle adult (40-60)?
    a. ____________________
    b. ____________________
    c. ____________________
    d. ____________________

42. According to Levinson's theory of adult development, life structure is centered around the interaction of three components. These are:
   a. ______________________________
   b. ______________________________
   c. ______________________________

   If something changes in one component, what happens to the life's structure?

   ____
   ____

43. Gould's theory of adult development revolves around what central theme?

   ____
   ____
   ____

Clinical Situations

Consider each question in relation to the clinical picture presented. Circle the correct answer.

Josh is an 18 month old toddler you are babysitting. He is bright, cheerful, and has an engaging smile -- except when he can't have his own way.

44. Josh's favorite word is "no". You understand this is a typical behavioral trait of the toddler. It is termed? *(Circle one)*
   A. Regression
   B. Negativism
   C. Pessimism
   D. Obstinateness
45. According to Havighurst, which of the following is the major developmental task of toddlerhood? *(Circle one)*
   A. Learning to control body wastes
   B. Learning sex differences
   C. Forming concepts and learning language
   D. Learning to distinguish right from wrong
46. Josh likes to explore his environment and is into everything constantly. His parents are most concerned. Knowing this, what role could you as a nurse assume that would be the most helpful for this family? *(Circle one)*
   A. Babysitter
   B. Confidante
   C. Teacher
   D. Bystander

47. Josh's mother expresses concern over his recent decrease in appetite. You could best explain this by which of the following statements? *(Circle one)*
    A. His growth rate has slowed and his appetite has followed suit.
    B. He doesn't like what you feed him.
    C. He is coming down with something.
    D. He must be teething.

Crystal is a 15 year old girl who has just been diagnosed with bulimia. She is being admitted to the adolescent unit and you have been assigned as her nurse.

48. Which of the following is the best definition of bulimia? *(Circle one)*
    A. Overeating
    B. Compulsive dieting to the point of self-starvation
    C. Binge eating followed by self-induced vomiting
    D. Uncontrolled diarrhea caused by overuse of laxative

49. While performing an admission physical on Crystal, you discover the following data: breast development has begun, axillary and pubic hair present, menstruation has begun, moderate degree of acne. Which stage of puberty would you classify Crystal as being in? *(Circle one)*
    A. Prepubescence
    B. Pubescence
    C. Postpubescence
    D. Pregnant

50. Crystal has also contemplated suicide. As a nurse you need to be aware of the fact that adolescent suicides as well as bulimia are clearly linked to which of the following? *(Circle one)*
    A. Disturbed family function
    B. Peer group pressure
    C. Teenage pregnancy
    D. STD's

51. Considering these facts, which of the following would be the most important nursing intervention you could accomplish under these circumstances? *(Circle one)*
    A. Get Crystal's entire family into therapy and involved with her care in order to facilitate the development of a healthy family relationship.
    B. Promote peer group activity and involvement in her care as peers have extraordinary influence at this age.
    C. Disseminate birth control information as she will most likely start to act out sexually considering the stress she is currently under.
    D. Help her to improve her skin condition (acne) in order to help foster a more positive self-image.

Sam and Sally are a young married couple in their early 20's who have approached you in preparation for their first child. Sally is four months pregnant.

52. Which trimester of the pregnancy is Sally in? *(Circle one)*
    A. First
    B. Second
    C. Third
    D. Fourth
53. What is a major psychosocial task for this trimester of pregnancy? *(Circle one)*
    A. Accepting the pregnancy
    B. Assuming responsibility for fetal well-being
    C. Performing maternal tasks in preparation for the infant
    D. Actively preparing for the labor and delivery process
54. Sally asks on her visit, "What does my baby look like now?" Which of the following descriptions would be appropriate? *(Circle one)*
    A. It weighs about one ounce and is about three inches long. You can tell if it is a boy or girl.
    B. The baby's skull is fully formed now but it has little subcutaneous fat.
    C. The eyes, mouth, and nose as well as the fingers and toes are formed and easily distinguished. You can tell which sex it is and it is about 6-10 inches long and weighs about seven ounces.
    D. It is covered with fine, downy hair. The fingers and toes are distinct and it would weigh about one and one-fourth pounds and be about fourteen inches long.
55. Sally asks, "If my baby were born now, would he live?" How would you respond?

    ____

    ____

56. Sally is concerned about the effect her pregnancy will have on her body. List some of the major physiologic changes Sally should be prepared to experience in the next few months.

    ____

    ____

    ____

    ____

    ____

    ____

57. Sam, being the prospective father, also has needs and concerns. List some of the areas that should be assessed with him so he can become an active and involved participant in the pregnancy.

    ____

    ____

    ____

    ____

    ____

    ____

58. Sam and Sally, being young adults, are in a time of relatively good health in their lives. However, physical and emotional problems can erupt often due to the hazards of life style choices made. List some of the specific problems that this couple might encounter and what the nurse's role might be to help them deal with it?

____

____

____

____

Roger and Hermine are a middle-aged couple. She is 45 and he is 47. They have just celebrated the event of their last teenager leaving for college.

59. Hermine is concerned with the amount of time she now has on her hands, and the overwhelming desire to "pick up" where she left off years ago when she gave up an aspiring business career to get married. She wants to go back to school. Hermine could be described as undergoing a *(Circle one)*
    A. Role Transition
    B. Situational Crisis
    C. Change of Life
    D. Midlife Crisis

60. Hermine will probably soon go through menopause. Which of the following best describes this phenomena? *(Circle one)*
    A. A gradual decrease in ovarian function with a depletion of estrogen and progesterone.
    B. A gradual loss in sexual appetite and functions.
    C. A gradual decline in ovarian function and sexual potency, but still capable of reproduction.
    D. No physiologic changes -- only complaints of psychological problems, ie. mood swings, fatigue, and depression

61. Roger at some time during this period will also undergo a similar process known as ________.

62. What advice would you give this couple for maintaining their health during this period of life -- age 40-60?

____

____

____

____

Additional Enrichment Activities

1. Obtain a recommended schedule of immunizations through childhood from a community health department, well-child clinic, hospital, or doctor's office. Keep it handy for reference.
2. Visit a Sunday school or vacation Bible school group. Observe several classes at various ages. Talk with the children about their beliefs in God. Compare your findings to Fowler's phases.
3. Invite a speech therapist to come to your class to discuss normal language development in children.
4. Visit a prenatal clinic or obstetrician's office. Talk with some of the women about their pregnancy. Compare your findings to the expected developmental tasks of the pregnant woman and the young adult female between 20 and 30.
5. Visit a newborn nursery. Observe the infants. Talk with the nurses about newborn characteristics and personalities. What concerns do new parents seem to have?
6. Visit a children's hospital/unit. Interview some of the children. See how they feel about being hospitalized. Compare and contrast the different ages. Relate their feelings with their appropriate level of growth and development. Observe play activities.
7. Read one of T. Berry Brazelton's books:
   Infants and Mothers, Delacorte Press, 1969, New York
   Toddlers and Parents, Delacorte Press, 1974
8. Assist in a screening clinic at a mall or with a neighborhood group or health center. Talk with the people who come about their health practices. Try to get a sample from all age groups to compare and contrast.

Suggested Readings

Allan JD: Identifications of health risks in young adult populations. J Community Health Nursing 4(1):223-33, 1987

Anderson CJ: Integration of the Brazelton Neonatal Assessment Scale into routine neonatal nursing care. Issues in Comprehensive Pediatric Nursing 9(5):341-51, 1986

Birchfield ME: Illness and children in a preschool center. Maternal Child Nurse J. 15(3):187-97, 1986

Brazelton T: To Listen to a Child, Reading, Mass: Addison-Wesley, 1984

Cantwell DP et al: Attention deficit disorders. Nurse Practitioner 12(7):38, 1987

Cherry BS et al: Changing concepts of childhood in society. Pediatric Nursing 12(6):421-4, 1986

Koniak-Griffin D: Developmental assessment with the Denver Developmental Screening Test: an effective approach for clinical instruction and performance evaluation, J. Pediatric Nursing 2(2): 1987

Panzarine S, et al: Adolsecent health care. J Nursing Education 27(6):276-280, 1988

Ryan P: Strategies for motivation life-style change. J. Cardiovascular Nursing 1(4):54-66, 1987

Rutledge DN: Factors related to women's practice of breast self-examination. Nursing Research 36(2):268-72, 1987

Stanford J: Testicular self-examination: teaching, learning and practice. J. Adv Nursing 12(1):13-9, 1987

Steele SM: Assessing developmental delays in presechool children. J Pediatric Health Care 2(3):141-5, 1988

Yoos L: Chronic childhood illnesses: Developmental issues. Pediatric Nursing 13(1):25-28, 1987

Computer Assisted Instruction

Developmental Concepts: Nursing applications in the ambulatory setting. Medi-Sim, Inc.

Chapter 12
The Older Adult

The focus of Chapter 12, Fundamentals of Nursing (Taylor, 1988) is on providing the learner with knowledge of the concepts of growth and development as they relate to the older adult.

After studying this chapter and completing the associated workbook exercises the student should be able to

- Define key terms used in the chapter.
- Describe common myths and stereotypes that perpetuate ageism.
- Gain awareness of own feelings and attitudes toward the aging process and the older adult.
- Compare physiologic and functional changes that occur with normal aging.
- Discuss developmental tasks of the older adult, as described by Erikson and Havighurst.
- Discuss nursing implications concerning the continued growth and development of the elderly client.
- List family and community resources that can be utilized to maintain the health and independence of the elderly client.

Key Terms Chapter 12

You will want to become familiar with the meaning of the following key terms used in this chapter.

ageism
alternative care
Alzheimer's disease
cognition
dementia
ego-integrity versus despair
frail-old
functional health
gerontic nursing
gerontology
iatrogenic
life review or reminiscence
old-old
older adult
presbycusis
reality orientation
social isolation
sundowning syndrome

Case Study Short Answer

Karen is a home health nurse. Mr. Williams, age 74, is one of her patients. By interviewing him and his son, she learns that he has been widowed for two years. He is hard of hearing and suffers from congestive heart failure, but he feels fairly well. The congestive heart failure is controlled by medication as long as he restricts his activity level. His son thinks he needs to enter a nursing home since Mr. Williams has never cooked nor kept house for himself. His wife always took care of him when she was alive. Mr. Williams insists, however, that he can manage to stay home with his dog and, in fact, has been doing just that. He uses canned food for his meals or occasionally goes to the local hamburger stand.

1. Because of his hearing problems, what should Karen do to facilitate communication with him?

____

____

____

____

2. When Karen visits Mr. Williams, she helps him organize a meal and his medications. She finds herself becoming frustrated when trying to explain what she has done. She keeps having to explain over and over to him. What must she remember about cognition and speed of processing when working with the elderly?

3. Even though Mr. Williams' house is very dusty, dishes are dirty, clothes are strewn around and weeds grow in his yard, he insists he can stay home and take care of himself. He is alone except when he walks to the corner McDonald's and when his son takes him out about once a month. The only constant companion he has is his dog. According to Havighurst, which developmental tasks is he meeting and which is he not meeting?

4. According to Erik Erikson's developmental stages, in which stage is Mr. Williams? Karen spends about an hour with Mr. Williams each time she is there, listening to him talk about his life as an electrician and about his life with his wife. In what way does her listening facilitate his favorable resolution of Erikson's stage?

5. Karen wants to help Mr. Williams meet his developmental tasks. What community agencies are there available in your community to help elderly such as Mr. Williams?

Additional Enrichment Activities

1. Visit an elderly relative, friend or neighbor. Encourage them to talk about their current life style. Find out what they look forward to in their life now. What gives them the greatest satisfaction? What activities do they enjoy the most? How does their current health limit them? What is their biggest frustration about aging?
2. After interviewing one or more ill elderly, see if you can decide if those persons have met Havighurst's developmental tasks for the elderly. What is their resolution of the Erikson stage they are in?

3. Try communicating with a classmate with some of the sensory alterations of the elderly. Crinkle a long piece of clear plastic wrap and cover your eyes with this, tying it behind your head. Put cotton balls in your ears. Place gloves on your hands. Try to talk normally to your friend. How does this affect your communication? Try eating a cookie with your gloved hands. What happens?

Suggested Readings

Billig N:To be old and sad: understanding depression in the elderly. Lexington, Mass., Lexington Books, 1987.

Burggraf V, Stomley M: Nursing the elderly. Philadelphia, Pa, JB Lippincott Company, 1988

Eliopoulos C: Care of the elderly. Philadelphia, Pa, JB Lippincott Company, 1988

Kohut JJ, Fleishman JL: Reality Orientation for the Elderly, (3rd ed). Oradell, New Jersey, Medical Economics Books, 1987

Speake DL: Health promotion in the well elderly. Health Values 11(6):25-30, 1987

Schultz PR, et al: Assessing community health needs of elderly populations: comparison of three strategies. J Advances in Nursing 13(2)193-202, 1988

Strumpf NE: A new age for elderly care. Nursing & Health Care 8(8):444-48, 1987

Wood WG, Strong R: Geriatric Clinical Pharmacokinetics. Raven Press, New York, 1985

Computer Assisted Instruction

Nursing Care of the Client with Alzheimer's Disease. Medi-Sim, Inc.

Chapter 13
Loss, Grief, and Death

The nurse is a key person in the care of both the client who is dying and the family, regardless of whether the client is at home or in a health care agency. This chapter of Fundamentals of Nursing (Taylor, 1988) provides the learner with opportunity to understand the phases of grieving and dying and become aware of one's own feelings about death. After studying this chapter, the learner should be able to

- Define key terms used in the chapter.
- Differentiate the types of loss.
- Describe the grief process and the stages of grief.
- Outline physiologic and psychologic care of a dying client.
- Identify ethical/legal issues concerning death.
- List the clinical signs of approaching death.
- Outline nursing responsibilities following death.
- Discuss the role of the nurse in caring for a client's family.

Key Terms Chapter 13

actual loss	*hospice*
anticipatory loss	*loss*
bereavement	*mourning*
death	*perceived loss*
dysfunctional grief	*physical loss*
grief	*psychologic loss*
grieving	*terminal illness*

Key Terms Match

Match the terms with the appropriate definitions.

Terms:

a. actual loss
b. anticipatory loss
c. bereavement
d. death
e. dysfunctional grief
f. loss
g. mourning
h. perceived loss
i. physical loss
j. psychological loss

Definitions:

1. ____ Irreversible cessation of circulatory and respiratory functions.
2. ____ Loss and grief behavior displayed for a loss yet to take place.
3. ____ Felt by an individual, but intangible to others, ie. youth, financial independence, etc.
4. ____ A physical or psychological loss recognized by others as well as by the person.
5. ____ Period of acceptance of loss and grief.
6. ____ An actual loss caused by altered self-image or inabilities.
7. ____ Abnormal, distorted or prolonged grief.
8. ____ A state of grieving during which an individual goes through grief reaction.
9. ____ Occurs when a valued person, object, or situation is changed or inaccessible.
10. ____ Actual loss of a body part or function.

True and False

Indicate whether the statement below is TRUE or FALSE

11. ____ Anticipatory loss is dysfunctional.
12. ____ In inhibited grief, the individual suppresses feelings of grief, and may manifest somatic symptoms.
13. ____ Normal grief is never delayed.
14. ____ Terminal care is concerned with the control of symptoms instead of with the control of disease.
15. ____ Abbreviated grief is dysfunctional.
16. ____ That nothing can be done to arrest the spread of tumor means that there is nothing to be done at all.

Additional Enrichment Activities

1. Locate a Holmes Readjustment Rating Scale. Identify life changes you might encounter regularly in your nursing practice. In a small group discuss why it is important to acknowledge and respond appropriately to these losses within medical settings.
2. List as many losses as you can imagine an elderly person might experience.
3. Identify a client that you are reasonably sure is grieving. Acknowledge the loss to the client and facilitate the expression of feelings.
4. Practice the sharing of feelings and concerns with another health care team member.

SUGGESTED READINGS

Archer DN et al: Sorrow has many faces: helping families cope with grief. Nursing 18(5):43-45, 1988

Boxwell AO: Geriatric suicide: the preventable death. Nursing Practice 13(6):10-11, 15, 18-19, 1988

Caplan H: It's time we helped patients die. RN 50(11):44-48, 1987

Castiglia PT: Death of a parent. J Health Care 2(3):157-159, 1988

Darden J: Dying at home. AD Nurse 3(1):21-22, 1988

Degner LF, et al: Preparing nurses for care of the dying: a longitudinal study. Cancer Nursing 11(3)1:60-169, 1988

Farnham R: Grief work with mothers of retarded children in a group. Issues in Mental Health Nursing 9(1):73-82, 1988

Gass KA: Coping strategies of widows. J Gerontological Nursing 12(8):29-33, 1987

Garrett JE: Multiple losses in older adults. J Gerontological Nursing 13(8):8-12, 1987

Greer S: Children grieve too. RN 51(8):19-21, 1988

Hutri MH: A quick reference table of interventions to assist families to cope with loss or neonatal death. Birth 15(1):33-35, 1988

Jezierski MB: We hurt too...nurses do experience pain. Nursing 18(4):160, 1988

Jones MB, et al: Nursing interventions with continuing loss. Focus on Critical Care 15(3):26-30, 1988

Lovell B: Sharing the death of a parent. Nursing Times 83(42):36-39, 1987

Melia K: An easy death?...active euthanasia. Nursing Times 84(8):46-48, 1988

Oerlemans-Bunn M: On being gay, single and bereaved. AJN 88(4):472-476, 1988

Petix M: Explaining death to school-age children. Pediatric Nursing 13(6):394-396, 1987

Unit IV
Nursing Process

Each of the five steps of nursing process are discussed in Unit IV: assessing, diagnosing, planning, implementing, and evaluating. Following an overview of the nursing process in Chapter 14, the learner is provided with additional information necessary for the beginning application of the nursing process in client care.

Chapter 14
Introduction to Nursing Process

Nurses are responsible for a unique dimension of health care, "the diagnosis and treatment of human response to actual or potential health problems" (American Nurses' Association, 1980). The nursing process is the systematic method that directs the activities of the nurse in providing client care in a variety of situations.

After studying this chapter of Fundamentals of Nursing (Taylor, 1988) and completing the associated workbook exercises, the student should be able to

- Define key terms used in the chapter.
- Describe the historic evolution of the nursing process.
- Describe the nursing process and each of its five steps.
- List three client and three nursing benefits of using the nursing process correctly.

Key Terms Chapter 14

assessing
diagnosing
evaluating
implementing
intuitive problem solving
nursing process
planning
scientific method
trial-and-error problem solving

Nursing Process

Match the letters A, B, C, D, and E with the correct statements. More than one letter may be required for some statements.

1. ____ Establishes priorities
2. ____ Involves continued data collection
3. ____ Identifies client strengths
4. ____ Establishes the data base
5. ____ Involves executing and documenting of care
6. ____ Validates data and nursing diagnoses
7. ____ Modifies the plan of care
8. ____ Writes client goals
9. ____ Identifies client health problems
10. ____ Measures client's achievement of goals
11. ____ Carries out the plan of care
12. ____ Interprets and analyzes data

A. Assessing
B. Diagnosing
C Planning
D. Implementing
E. Evaluating

Experiential Learning Activities

1. The scientific method of problem solving is a skill which is learned and applied not only to nursing but to daily living. Think of a problem area in your own life (think of something not health related). Discuss how you would approach the problem using the five steps of the problem-solving or nursing process.

Suggested Readings

Buchanan BF: Conceptual models: an assessment framework. J Nursing Administration 17(10):22-6, 1987
Carlson C, et al: Nursing process how to's. AD Nurse 2(1):24-7, 1987
Henderson V: Nursing process, a critique. Holistic Nursing Practice 1(3):7-1, 1987
Gerrity PL: Perception in nursing: The value of intuition. Holistic Nursing Practice 1(3):63-71, 1987

Computer Assisted Instruction

The Nursing Process. Medi-Sim, Inc.
Nursing Process Concepts and Skills. J.B. Lippincott Company

Suggested Readings

Chapter 15
Assessing

The systematic and continuous collection, validation, and communication of client data is explored in Chapter 15 (Taylor, 1988) and provides the learner with concepts essential to obtaining a comprehensive data base for client care. Concepts essential to interviewing for a client history and performing a nursing examination are presented as well as methods for verifying data and recording data.
After studying this chapter and completing the associated workbook exercises, the learner should be able to

- Define key terms used in the chapter.
- Describe the purposes of the initial comprehensive nursing assessment and of ongoing nursing assessments.
- Differentiate a nursing assessment from a medical assessment.
- Differentiate objective and subjective data.
- Describe the purposes of nursing observation, interview, and examination.
- Obtain a nursing history using effective interviewing techniques.
- Identify five sources of client data useful to the nurse.
- Differentiate comprehensive admission assessments from focused assessments.
- Plan client assessments by identifying assessment priorities and structuring the data to be collected systematically.
- Identify common problems encountered in data collection noting their possible cause and etiology.
- Explain when data need to be validated and several ways to accomplish this.
- Describe the importance of knowing when to report significant client data and the importance of proper documentation.
- Obtain complete, accurate, relevant, and factual client data.

Key Terms Chapter 15

assessing
data
data base
interview
nursing examination
nursing history
objective data
observation
subjective data
validation

Completion

Complete the following statements.

1. The second phase of the interview is the ______________
2. The nurse interviews the client to obtain a __________ _______
3. Assessments should be______________ to assure comprehensive data collection.
4. Nursing assessments are modified according to the ______________ needs of the client.
5. The admission data base is also called ______________.
6. Assessments which define underlying pathology are ______________.
7. To confirm or verify data is also referred to as to ______________ data.
8. A systematic collection of client data is known as ______________.
9. Information perceived only by the client is called ______________.
10. The fourth phase of the interview is ______________.
11. The recording of client data is referred to as ______________.
12. Information perceived by the senses is called ______________.
13. Conscious and deliberate use of the senses to collect data is known as ______

Experiential Learning Activity

Most health care institutions have either developed their own method of structuring an assessment, or they have adopted a more formal framework based on a health related theory. No matter what the framework for the assessment tool, structuring is important in order to assist in organizing the data and assuring a comprehensive assessment. Get together with about 3 of your fellow students and each of you select a different health-care institution in your community. Visit the agency and ask for a copy of their admission assessment tool. Then, compare and contrast the tool with those collected by other members in your group. See if you can identify a specific theory upon which the assessment form is based (i.e. Maslow's hierarchy of needs, Gordon's eleven functional health patterns). Identify aspects of the tools which you believe are helpful and those which you might change.

Suggested Readings

Assessing Your Patients: Nursing Photobook. Horsham, PA, Nursing Intermed Communications, Inc., 1980

Barker P: Assembling the pieces...assessment is like a jigsaw puzzle. Nursing Times 83 (47):67-68, 1987

Brown MD: Functional assessment of the elderly. Gerontological Nursing 14(5):131-17, 1988

Burnard P: Meaningful dialogue...elements that comprise a therapeutic conversation. Nursing Times 83(20):42-45, 1987

Derdiarian A: A valid profession needs valid diagnoses. Nursing and Health Care 9(3): 136-140, 1988

Hanna DV et al: Assessment + diagnosis = careplanning: a tool for coordination. Nursing Management 18(11): 106-109, 1987

Seyster K: A lesson in therapeutic relationship. Imprint. September-October, 34(3): 56-57, 1987

Spillane RN: Assessment: getting the patient's point of view -- early. Nursing Management 18(5): 20, 22, 24, 1987

Williams K: World view and the facilitation of wholeness. Holistic Nursing Practice 18(5), 1987

Computer Assisted Instruction

Nursing Process Concepts and Skills, JB Lippincott Company

Nursing Process, Medi-Sim, Inc.

Chapter 16
Diagnosing

The unique focus of nursing diagnoses is the subject of Chapter 16 in Fundamentals of Nursing (Taylor, 1988). While a brief history of the evolution of nursing diagnoses was given in Chapter 14, the purpose of Chapter 16 is to assist the learner to identify (1) actual and potential problems in the way the client responds to health or illness, (2) factors contributing to or causing the above problems (etiologies), and (3) strengths the client can draw on to prevent or resolve the problem.

After studying this chapter and completing the associated workbook exercises, the learner should be able to

- Define key terms used in the chapter.
- Describe the term nursing diagnosis, distinguishing it from a collaborative problem and a medical diagnosis.
- Describe the four steps involved in data interpretation and analysis.
- Use the guidelines for writing nursing diagnoses when developing diagnostic statements.
- List four advantages of using the NANDA approved list of nursing diagnoses.
- Describe means to validate nursing diagnoses.
- Develop a prioritized list of nursing diagnoses using identifiable criteria.
- Describe the benefits and limitations of nursing diagnoses.

Key Terms Chapter 16

Prior to beginning the workbook exercises associated with Chapter 16 of Fundamentals of Nursing, the learner will want to become familiar with the following key terms

collaborative problem
cue
data cluster
diagnosing
health problem
medical diagnosis
nursing diagnosis
actual problems
possible problems
potential problems

Nursing Diagnoses : Match

From the nursing diagnoses written below, identify the error/s in each by placing the letter of the Common Error/s in the list provided which describes what is wrong with the diagnosis statement. Some of the diagnoses are correctly written; if so, indicate by writing *correct* in the space provided.

Common Errors
A. Identifying responses not necessarily unhealthy
B. Using legally inadvisable language
C. Including value judgments
D. Including medical diagnoses

Nursing Diagnoses
1. ____ Potential for Injury r/t absence of restraints and side rails
2. ____ Nutrition, Alteration in: Less Than Body Requirements r/t loss of appetite
3. ____ Grieving r/t loss of breast
4. ____ Powerlessness r/t poor family support system
5. ____ Anxiety: mild r/t changing life-style/diet
6. ____ Ineffective Airway Clearance r/t weak cough
7. ____ Ineffective Breathing Patterns r/t emphysema
8. ____ Potential for Violence r/t history of violent behavior
9. ____ Alteration in Bowel Elimination: Constipation r/t cancer of the bowel
10. ____ Anxiety: severe r/t impaired verbal communication

Common Errors

E. Both clauses say the same thing
F. Reversing the clauses
G. Identifying problems as signs and symptoms
H. Identifying problems/etiologies that cannot be altered

Nursing Diagnoses

11. ____ Sleep Pattern Disturbance r/t insomnia
12. ____ Nausea and vomiting r/t medication side effects
13. ____ Knowledge Deficit r/t noncompliance with diet
14. ____ Inadequate parenting r/t ineffective family coping
15. ____ Dysfunctional Grieving r/t inability to accept loss of breast
16. ____ Alteration in Comfort r/t pain in abdomen
17. ____ Disturbance in Self-concept r/t sexual dysfunction
18. ____ Confusion r/t Alteration in thought processes
19. ____ Impaired Physical Mobility: amputation left leg r/t gangrene
20. ____ Ineffective Individual Coping r/t drug abuse
21. ____ Self-care Deficit: bathing/hygiene r/t right-sided paralysis
22. ____ Fear: of rejection r/t social isolation
23. ____ Nutrition, Alteration in: More Than Body Requirements r/t obesity
24. ____ Weakness r/t activity intolerance
25. ____ Inadequate resources r/t knowledge deficit regarding stress management

Experiential Learning Activities

Utilizing a health care agency/institution in your community, explore the use of nursing diagnoses in that particular hospital, nursing home, etc. Compare and contrast writing nursing diagnoses in different settings within that institution such as a medical-surgical unit versus emergency room or labor and delivery. If you select a nursing home, you might compare and contrast nursing diagnoses between a skilled unit versus an independent living type of unit. Write down five or six nursing diagnoses you find in the Nursing Kardex and use the guidelines for writing nursing diagnoses to critique them.

Suggested Readings

Giger JB, et al: Roy Adaptation Model: ICU application. D Critical Care Ns 6(4):215-24, 1987

Gordon M: Implementation of Nsg Dx: an overview. Nursing Clinics North Am 22(4): 875-880, 1987

Halloran EJ, et al: Case-mix: Matching patient need with nursing resources. Nursing diagnosis-based patient classification system. Nursing Management 18(3):27-30, 1987

Maas ML: Nursing diagnosis in a professional model of nursing: Keystone for effective nursing administration. J Nursing Administration 16(12):39-42, 1987

MacLeod F, et al: Solving the nursery care plan dilemma: nursing diagnosis makes the difference. J Nursing Staff Development 4(2):70-3, 1988

Roberts S: The future marriage between diagnosis related groups and nursing diagnosis related groups. Critical Care Nursing Quarterly 9(4):70-82, 1987

Introduction to nursing diagnosis. Nursing Process Concepts and Skills Series. JB Lippincott Company

Computer Assisted Instruction

Nursing Process Concepts and Skills, JB Lippincott Company

Nursing Process, Medi-Sim, Inc.

Chapter 17
Planning

Planning, the third phase of nursing process, is approached by the authors of Fundamentals of Nursing (Taylor, 1988) as the development of a holistic, individualized plan of nursing care collaboratively arrived at between the client/family and the nurse.
After studying this chapter and completing the associated workbook exercises, the learner should be able to

- Define key terms used in the chapter.
- Describe the purpose and benefits of planning.
- Identify three elements of comprehensive planning.
- Prioritize client health problems and nursing responses.
- Describe how client goals and nursing orders are derived from nursing diagnoses.
- Develop a plan of nursing care with properly constructed goals and related nursing orders.
- Use criteria to evaluate planning skills.
- Describe five common problems related to planning, their possible causes, and remedies.

Key Terms Chapter 17

The learner will find it beneficial to become familiar with the key terms used in the chapter prior to attempting the workbook exercises.

client goal (objective, outcome)
criteria
discharge planning
goal
Kardex care plan
nursing care plan
nursing measure
nursing order
planning
priority setting
standardized care plan

Client Goals Categorized

Categorize the following goals according to the type of change they describe for the client.

- Cognitive
- Psychomotor
- Affective

1. ________ By 2/7 client will list foods high in sodium
2. ________ By 2/7 client will trust nurse enough to volunteer expression of feelings
3. ________ By 2/7 client correctly demonstrates subQ injections using normal saline
4. ________ By 6/12 client correctly demonstrates application of wet to dry dressing on leg ulcer
5. ________ By 6/12 Client will list 3 benefits of psychotherapy

Writing Goal Statements

For each of the four goal statements below label the parts of the statement as being either:

A. Subject
B. Verb
C. Criteria, or
D. Special Conditions, if any.

Some of the answers are provided for you, for instance, in #6 *Client* is *A*, the subject.

6. *Client correctly demonstrates application of wet to dry dressing on leg ulcer by 6/12.*
   _A_ ______ __________ ____.
7. *Client will list three benefits of psychotherapy by 6/12*
   _____ ______ ______________________________.
8. *At next visit, client correctly demonstrates relaxation exercises.*
   _________ ____ __C__ _________ __C__________.
9. *Prior to discharge, client ambulates independently in hallway, using crutches.*
   ____________ ____ _______ __________________ __________.

Guidelines for Selecting Nursing Actions

List 3 guidelines the nurse can use when selecting nursing measures from available options.

10. ____
11. ____
12. ____

Writing Nursing Orders

The set of nursing orders to help a client meet a goal must be comprehensive. Comprehensive nursing orders include:

13. ___________ that need to be made and how often.
14. What ________ ________ need to be done and when.
15. ____________________, _______, and advocacy needs of clients.
16. Priorities for ___________________________ assessment.

Nursing Kardex

List the three types of information usually found on an institutional care plan (Kardex). Nursing care related to:

17. ____
18. ____
19. ____

For a client with a nursing diagnosis of sleep pattern disburbance r/t pain and anxiety, match the items below to the correct side of the nursing diagnosis table.

	Sleep pattern disturbance	r/t pain and anxiety
20. Give backrub at 9:00 p.m.		
21. Client will fall asleep by 10:00 p.m. by 5/1		
22. Assess degree of client's pain, using a 1-5 pain rating scale		
23. Client will report feeling rested in the a.m. on 5/1		
24. Position client for minimal strain on incision at bedtime		

Additional Enrichment Activities

1. Look at the care plans (Kardex) in the agency where you are assigned for clinical laboratory experiences.
    a. Where are the nursing care plans kept (eg. notebook, Kardex)
    b. Are they written in ink?
    c. Are standardized care plans used? How?
    d. Do they contain information about nursing care related to:
        (1) basic human needs?
        (2) nursing diagnoses?
        (3) the medical plan of care?
            (Give examples of these types of information)
2. While you are in the clinical agency, copy three goals from a patient care plan to discuss with your study group.
    a. Do the goals contain subject, verb and criteria?
    b. Are they short-term or long-term?
    c. Are they measurable?
    d. What would you do to improve them?

Suggested Readings

Bader MM: Nursing care behaviors that predict patient satisfaction. J Nursing Quality Assurance 2(3): 11-17, 1988

Cobb SC et al: Nursing rounds: idea to reality. Oncology nursing forum. January-February 15(1): 23-27, 1988

George JE et al: Standardized care plans: legal implications. J of Emergency Nursing 14(3):183-184

McElroy D et al: Writing a better patient care plan. Nursing 18(2):50-51

McLeod F et al: Solving the nursing care plan dilemma: Nursing diagnosis makes the difference. J of Nursing Staff Development Spring, 4(2): 70-73, 1988

Scher BB: Are checklists replacing good care? Nurse 18(1):47 1988

Shine MS: Discharge planning for the elderly patient in the acute care setting. Nursing Clinics of North America 18:409, 1983

Wicker P: Putting ideas into practice. Senior Nurse 7(4):22-24, 1987

Wright S: Primary nursing: patient-centered practice. Nursing Times 83(38): 24-27

Zander K: Nursing case management: Strategic management of cost and quality outcomes. J Nursing administration 18(5): 23-30, 1988

Computer Assisted Instruction

Nursing Process Concepts and Skills. JB Lippincott Company

Nursing Process, Medi-Sim, Inc.

Chapter 18
Implementing/Documenting

The focus of chapter 18 of the Taylor (1988) Fundamentals of Nursing textbook is to provide the learner with opportunities to explore the phase of the nursing process where the nursing actions developed during the planning step are carried out.
After studying this chapter, and completing the associated workbook exercises, the learner should be able to

- Define key terms used in the chapter.
- Distinguish independent, interdependent or collaborative, and dependent nursing interventions.
- Use intellectual, interpersonal, and technical skills to implement a plan of nursing care.
- Describe six variables that influence the way a plan of care is implemented.
- Use seven guidelines for implementation.
- Use ongoing data collection to direct revision of the plan of care.
- Compare and contrast different documentation systems: source-oriented record, problem-oriented record, and computer record.
- Document nursing interventions completely, accurately, concisely, and factually.
- Describe nursing's role in communicating with other health-care professionals by reporting, conferring, and referring.

Key Terms Chapter 18

Prior to attempting the workbook exercises the learner will want to become familiar with the following key terms used in Chapter 18

change-of-shift report
dependent intervention
discharge summary
flow sheets
implementing
independent intervention
interdependent (collaborative) intervention
nursing actions (interventions, measures, strategies)
nursing care conference
nursing care round
problem-oriented record (POR)
progress notes
protocol
record
SOAP format
source-oriented record
standing order

Documentation with Abbreviations

Rewrite the following paragraph, using acceptable abbreviations where possible.

1. *Client has been out of bed twice this shift. Complains of mild pain in abdomen on ambulation, but no pallor or shortness of breath. Oxygen discontinued at 9:00 a.m. Homan's sign negative. Blood pressure, pulse and respirations are within normal limits. Abdomen soft, not distended; bowel sounds auscultated in all four quadrants. No bowel movement today. Reminded client of need to void in receptacle for measurement of intake and output.*

____

____

____

____

____

____

____

____

____

____

____

____

Communication Methods and their Disadvantages

2. Draw lines to match the methods of communication with their disadvantages. Each method may have more than one disadvantage. Some disadvantages may match more than one method.

<u>Method</u>

Face-to-Face Meeting

Telephone conversation

Written message

Audiotaped message

<u>Disadvantage</u>

a. Message usually cannot be validated with the sender

b. Ordinarily there is no permanent record for later use

c. No nonverbal message can be given

d. Both the sending and receiving persons must be available at the same time, in the same place

e. Only the tone of voice and voice inflections can be communicated

Implementation Guidelines

3. List and discuss three guidelines for successful implementation of the plan of care.

A. ____

B. ____

C. ____

Additional Enrichment Activities

1. Interview at least three R.N.s. Ask them to list for you the independent nursing functions they have performed so far during the shift. Share this information with your study group.
2. Attend either a change-of-shift report, a nursing care conference, or nursing rounds. What information is communicated? How is the information communicated?
3. Find out how computers are used in your clinical institution. Are there computers on the nursing unit? What are they used for? Who uses them?
4. Evaluate the nursing documentation in a client's chart. Base your evaluation on the "Guidelines for Documentation" on pp. 466-468 of your text. Copy a few examples (good or bad) to support your evaluation, and discuss them in class.

Suggested Readings

Bulechek GM, McCloskey JC: Nursing interventions: What they are and how to choose them. Holistic Nursing Practice 1(3):27-35, 1987

Cushing M: The legal side: Dealing with details. AJN 88(7):955-57

Irabenstein J: Nursing documentation during perinatal period. J Perinatal Neonatal Nursing 1(2):29-38, 1987

Kilpack V et al: Intershift report: oral communication using the nursing process. J Neuroscience Nursing 19(5):266-70, 1987

Nurses notes worth their weight in gold: Regan Report in Nursing Law 27(8):1, 1987

Computer Assisted Instruction

Nursing Process Concepts and Skills. J.B. Lippincott Company

Nursing Process, Medi-Sim, Inc.

Chapter 19
Evaluating

The unique focus of evaluation, the fifth step in the nursing process, is the subject of Chapter 19 in Fundamentals of Nursing (Taylor, 1988). During the evaluation phase of the nursing process the nurse measures the extent to which goals have been met; determines factors contributing to the client's success or failure; and either modifies, terminates, or continues with the plan of care as needed.

After studying Chapter 19 and completing the workbook exercises the learner should be able to

- Define key terms used in the chapter.
- Describe evaluation, its purpose, and relationship to other steps in the nursing process.
- Evaluate the client's achievement of goals specified in the plan of care.
- Manipulate factors contributing to the client's success or failure in goal achievement.
- Use the client's responses to the plan of care to modify the plan as needed.
- Explain the relationship between quality assurance programs and excellence in health care.

Key Terms Chapter 19

criteria
evaluating
nursing audit
  concurrent
  retrospective
outcome evaluation
quality assurance program
standard

Evaluation Standards and Criteria

Identify which of the following are evaluation "criteria" (C), and which are "standards" (S).

1. ____ Client will be able to walk length of the hall unassisted by 5/15.
2. ____ Upon completion of the EKG course, the nurse will be able to recognize common arrhythmias when they appear on a cardiac monitor.
3. ____ All patients in active labor will have continuous external fetal heart monitoring.
4. ____ The admission data base will be completed on all patients within 24 hours after admission to the unit.
5. ____ The student will be able to name and describe the steps of the nursing process by the end of the semester.

Factors Impacting on Quality of Nursing Care

The variables below may detract from quality nursing care. Discuss approaches a nurse might use to solve each of these problems.

6. Inadequate staffing -

____

____

____

7. Boredom, loss of interest in nursing -

____

____

____

8. Inadequate supplies -

____

____

____

Data Correlated to Type of Evaluation

For which type of evaluation can the following data be used: *structure*, *process* or *outcome*?

9. ________ Client able to walk to bathroom without pallor or shortness of breath.
10. ________ All charting entries are signed with nurse's first initial, last name and title.

11. ________ A head-to-toe assessment is charted on every patient at least once a day.
12. ________ Each primary nurse is assigned no more than 6 patients for a caseload.
13. ________ There are 7 fetal monitors in the labor and delivery area.
14. ________ No superficial redness or edema of extremities. Homan's sign negative.

Additional Enrichment Activities

1. In clinical, examine your client's care plan and chart.
   Where are the evaluative statements written?
   Do the evaluative statements:
      (1) indicate the client's progress toward meeting the goal and
      (2) give client data to support that conclusion?
   Are there evaluative statements made for every goal in the care plan?
2. Talk to the nurses in the agency where you have clinical.
   How many patients do they usually care for during a shift?
   Do they believe they can effectively care for this number of patients?
   How does this unit decide how many nurses are needed for each shift?
3. In your clinical agency, find the "Procedures" book on your unit.
   Make a list of six procedures to share in class.
   Find the "Policies" book; list six different policies.
   Compare your lists with those of your classmates.
   How are procedures different from policies?

Suggested Readings

Beyers M: Guest Editor Quality Assurance, Philadelphia, PA, Nursing Clinics North Am 23(3):613-679, 1987

Dirschel KM: A mandate for standards of care. Nursing Health and Care 7(1):27-29, 1986

Kanon RJ: Standards of nursing practice assessed through the application of the nursing process. Journal of Nursing Quality Assurance 1(2):72-8, 1987

Osinski E: Developing patient outcomes as a quality measure of nursing care. Nursing Management 18(10): 28-9, 1987

Computer Assisted Instruction

Evaluation of Nursing Interventions. Medi-Sim, Inc.

Nursing Process Concepts and Skills. J.B. Lippincott Company

Unit V
Roles Basic to Nursing Practice

Unit V provides content necessary to the caregiver role, e.g. communicator, teacher, counselor, leader, researcher, advocate. Nursing practice that is holistic and client-centered is based on an application of the knowledge and skills associated with these various roles.

Chapter 20 Communicator

One of the most significant roles of the nurse is that of communicator. The characteristics of the communication process are presented in Chapter 20 of Taylor Fundamentals of Nursing (1988). The communication skills nurses must possess in order to be effective caregivers are discussed.

After studying this chapter and completing the associated workbook pages, the learner should be able to

- Define key terms used in the chapter.
- Describe the communication process.
- List at least eight ways in which people communicate nonverbally.
- Describe the interrelationships between communication and the nursing process.
- Describe the phases of a helping relationship.
- Practice each of the effective communication techniques.
- Explain why the development of interpersonal skills is important for the nurse.
- Describe each of the ineffective communication techniques.
- Explain how to facilitate nurse-client interactions in special circumstances.

Key Terms Chapter 20

communication
empathy
helping relationship
interpersonal skills
interviewing techniques
language
nonverbal communication
rapport
relationship
semantics
therapeutic touch
verbal communication

Communication: True/False

Indicate whether the following statements are true or false.

1. ____ Communication requires at least two persons.
2. ____ Communication is influenced by the way people feel.
3. ____ The message can be assumed to mean what the sender intended it to mean.
4. ____ In true communication, one person only "sends" and the other only "receives."
5. ____ Verbal and nonverbal communication occur at the same time.
6. ____ Feedback is important in order to know if a message was received accurately.
7. ____ If the message is received accurately, the true meaning will also be known.

Communication and the Nursing Process

8. List examples of ways the nurse uses communication in each phase of the nursing process.
   a. data collection
   ____
   ____

   b. diagnosis
   ____
   ____

   c. planning
   ____
   ____

   d. implementation
   ____
   ____

   e. evaluation
   ____
   ____

9. List three characteristics of a helping (therapeutic) relationship.
   a. ____________________
   b. ____________________
   c. ____________________

10. Discuss ways in which the nurse can achieve termination of a relationship that will be satisfactory to both client and nurse.

____
____
____
____
____
____

Communication Match

Match the following dialogue examples with the correct interviewing technique.

Dialogue Examples:

11. ____ *Nurse:* What did your doctor tell you about taking your blood pressure medicine?

12. ____ *Nurse:* How long have you been taking blood pressure medicine?

13. ____ *Client:* There is no point in taking this medicine.
Nurse: Are you saying you don't feel any better when you take it?

14. ____ *Client:* My father had this same surgery 20 years ago and he was never the same afterwards. Maybe I won't be the same either.
Nurse: The same. . .

15. ____ *Nurse:* Let's see, did the nausea begin before or after you started taking the medicine for your heart?

Interviewing Techniques:

A. closed question/comment
B. validating question/comment
C. clarifying question/comment
D. reflective question/comment
E. sequencing question/comment
F. directing question/comment
G. open-ended question/comment

Communication Crossword Puzzle

Complete the crossword puzzle, using words describing ways we communicate.

Across

1.____ expresses very personal behavior, and is effective in expressing feelings.
2. Verbal communication uses ____.
3. ____ shows respect and a willingness to listen.
4. ____ are used extensively when people are speaking different languages.
5. Healthy people pay attention to details of ____ and grooming.

Down

1. The way a person holds his body.
2. Nonverbal communication.
3. ____ may mean anything from complete understanding to anger.
4. Nurses need to control their ____ expressions to a degree.
5. Crying, gasping and moaning are oral, but nonverbal
6. Same as touch.

Additional Enrichment Activities

1. After caring for a client in the clinical laboratory, analyze your relationship to see if it was social or therapeutic. Use the information on pp. 515-517 of your textbook as a guide.
2. After caring for a client in the clinical laboratory, assess how well you were able to control the factors discussed on pp. 529-530 of your textbook (objectives for the interaction, comfort, privacy, confidentiality, client focus, use of nursing observations, pacing, personal space). How did these factors affect your interactions with your client?
3. Observe as a classmate provides care. In what ways was touch used? How did the client respond?

Suggested Readings

Ashton E: A simple message: this nurse learned that the best communication often is unspoken. Nursing Life 8(2):21, 1988

Bond M: Assertive rights and body language. Nursing Times 84(11):67-70, 1988

Burand P: Four dimensions in counseling. Nursing Times 84(20):37-39, 1988

Cunliff PH: Communicating with children in the intensive care unit...triadic relationship of child/parent/nurse. Intensive Care Nursing 3(2):71-77, 1987

Cushnie P: Conflict: developing resolution skills AORN J 43(3):732-735, 1988

Garvin BJ et al: Confirming communication of nurses in interaction with physicians. J Nursing Education 27(4):161-166, 1988

Honeycutt JM et al: Impressions about communication styles and competence in nursing relationships. Communication Education 36(3)217-227, 1987

McAlvanab NF: Communication: a two-way street. Pediatric Nursing 14(2)140, 1988

Nichols FH et al: Are your group process skills up to par? Nursing and Health Care 9(4):204-208, 1988

Nielsen E et al: Television as a patient education tool: a review of its effectiveness. Patient Education and Counseling 11(1):3-16, 1988

Orlick S: The primacy of caring. American Journal of Nursing 88(3):318-19, 1988

Pearce J: The power of touch. Nursing Times 84(24):26-29, 1988

Rankin WW: Listening with the heart...to listen to a child. J Pediatric Nursing 3(2):127-129, 1988

Smeltzer CH: A method for discussing nursing issues. J Nursing Administration 18(3):4-5, 1988

Thomas DO: How to make your point on paper. RN 5(18):14,18, 1988

Chapter 21
Teacher/Counselor

Regardless of the setting, the nurse's role as teacher/counselor is an important aspect of providing nursing care. These roles are dependent upon how well the nurse applies communication skills in the process. The Fundamentals of Nursing text (Taylor, 1988) points out that the trends in health care have made the roles of teacher and counselor increasingly important.

After studying this chapter and completing the workbook exercises for Chapter 21, the learner should be able to

- Define key terms used in the chapter.
- Describe the teaching-learning process, including domains, developmental concerns, and specific principles.
- Describe what factors should be assessed for the learning process.
- Compose diagnoses for identified learning needs.
- Explain how to create a teaching plan for a client.
- Describe what is involved in implementing a teaching plan.
- Name three methods for evaluation of learning.
- Explain what should be included in the documentation of the teaching-learning process.
- Discuss the nurse's role as a counselor.
- Summarize how the nursing process is used to assist clients in problem solving.
- Describe how to use the counseling role to motivate a client toward health promotion.

Key Terms

Prior to attempting the workbook exercises, the learner should become familiar with the key terms used in the chapter.

affective learning
cognitive learning
contractual agreement
counseling
developmental crisis
formal teaching
informal teaching
learning
psychomotor learning
situational crisis
teaching

Teaching Role of the Nurse: Short Answer

1. Discuss reasons why it is more important than ever for nurses to improve the quality of their client teaching.

____

____

____

____

Define the following terms related to the teacher and counselor roles of the nurse.

2. teaching:

____

3. learning:

____

4. situational crisis:

____

5. developmental crisis:

____

Teaching/Learning :True / False

6. ____ Nurse-teachers do only one-to-one teaching.
7. ____ Learning is facilitated by the existence of a helping relationship.
8. ____ Sensory stimulation is detrimental to learning.
9. ____ New knowledge is better assimilated if it can be related to the client's past life experiences.

Teaching Assessment : Table Completion

Complete the table by explaining why it is important to assess a client for each of the factors prior to implementing a teaching plan.

Assessment Factor	Rationale for Assesssment
10. Developmental level	
11. Level of education	
12. Emotional health	
13. Self-image	
14. Culture	

Evaluation of Teaching

15. Discuss how nurses can evaluate their teaching.

Teaching Strategies : Matching

Match the teaching strategies in the list below with the examples of teaching episodes.

Teaching Strategies

A. demonstration
B. role playing
C. lecture
D. panel discussion
E. role modeling

Teaching Episodes

16. ____ The nurse chooses a low-calorie diet for herself when eating with an obese patient on a weight-loss program.
17. ____ Oral presentation of information to a large group of clients.
18. ____ Four parents of developmentally delayed children present information to a group of nursing students.
19. ____ A nurse bathes a newborn while the mother watches.
20. ____ One student pretends to be a patient, while the other student practices a nursing interview.

Counseling Completion

Fill in the blanks in the sentences below by choosing the correct answer from the list provided.

Correct Answers
long-term
short-term
situational
developmental
motivational

21. A client experiencing a ________________ crisis probably would need short-term counseling.
22. Long-term counseling would probably be used for a ______________ crisis.
23. ______________________ counseling focuses on the immediate problem.
24. ______________________ counseling may extend over months or years.
25. If a client is not interested in learning, ______________ counseling may be needed.

Learning Domains

When establishing learning objectives it is helpful to use verbs reflective of the learning domain. Place the verbs in the list below in the appropriate domain listed in the table.

<u>*Verb List*</u>	*chooses*	*explains*	*shares*
arranges	*constructs*	*helps*	*shows*
assembles	*defends*	*justifies*	*states*
categorizes	*defines*	*lists*	

26. Cognitive Domain	27. Affective Domain	28. Psychomotor Domain

29. Which of the verbs in the list above would be useful in writing goals for a client with following diagnoses?

a. *Knowledge deficit: side effects of Coumarin related to inexperience with anti-coagulant therapy* *Verb:* __________________________

b. *Knowledge deficit: bathing newborn related to inexperience (first baby)* Verb: __________________________

c. *Knowledge deficit: low calorie diet related to lack of motivation to lose weight* Verb: _______________________

Additional Learning Activities

1. Suppose you have a client who needs specialized or intense counseling that you are unable to provide. Make a list of the agencies in your area to which you could refer the client. You might begin by looking in the telephone book.
2. Find out how much it costs in your area to have individual and group counseling. What agencies are available for clients with limited funds?
3. Identify the teaching needs of a client you care for in clinical laboratory. Write a teaching plan to meet those needs. Be sure to build in a method of evaluation.

Suggested Readings

Cox CL: The health self-determinism index. Nursing Research 34(3):177-83, 1985

Palmer ME, Deck ES: Teaching your patients to assert their rights. American Journal of Nursing 87(5):650-54, 1987

Robinson M: Patient advocacy and the nurse: Is there a conflict of interest? Nursing Forum 22(2):58-63, 1985

Computer Assisted Instruction

Nursing Process Concepts and Skills. "Introduction to Behavioral Objectives." JB Lippincott Company

Chapter 22
Leader/Research/Advocate

The relationship between leadership, research, and advocacy are explored in this chapter of Fundamentals of Nursing (Taylor, 1988).
After studying this chapter and completing the workbook exercises, the learner should be able to

- Define key terms used in the chapter.
- Identify the qualities of a good leader.
- Describe the three styles of leadership.
- Summarize the eight steps in the process of change.
- List the four functions of a nurse manager.
- Describe how the nurse uses leadership abilities for the benefit of the client, the nursing team, the nursing profession, and society.
- Give an example of mentorship in nursing.
- State one characteristic that differentiates a profession from an occupation.
- Describe an example of a nursing intervention based on authoritative knowledge.
- Describe a nursing intervention based on scientific knowledge.
- Discuss the significance of the Patient's Bill of Rights.
- Compare assertive behavior with aggressive behavior.
- Describe the nurse advocate's role in situations requiring ethical decisions.

Key Terms Chapter 22

The learner will want to become familiar with the following key terms used in Chapter 22 prior to attempting the workbook exercises.

advocacy
assertiveness
authoritative knowledge
change
change agent
group process
leadership
- *autocratic leadership*
- *democratic leadership*
- *laissez-faire leadership*

mentorship
objectivity
planned change
professionalism
readiness
scientific knowledge
traditional knowledge
variables
- *dependent variables*
- *extraneous variables*
- *independent variables*

Leader Characteristics

List five characteristics which you possess that you think would make you a good leader.

1. ______________________________
2. ______________________________
3. ______________________________
4. ______________________________
5. ______________________________

Leadership Style: Match

Match the situations below with the correct leadership style (A, B, C).

Leadership Style

A. Democratic
B. Autocratic
C. Laissez-faire

6. _____ As head nurse, you notice a personality problem between two of your staff members. Both are very good nurses, and usually get along well. Patient care is not suffering, and you decide to let the two work it out for themselves.
7. _____ The fire alarm in the hospital has just sounded. There is a fire on the floor below yours. You immediately gather the unit staff and issue instructions for patient evacuation according to hospital policy.

8. ____ Your staff is resisting a proposed change on your unit. The change will be beneficial to both patients and staff. You call a staff meeting, explain the change, the benefits, and why it is necessary. You then ask your staff if they have any ideas that will help facilitate the change.

9. ____ Your patient for the day, Mr. Thurston, has been hospitalized repeatedly for non-compliance with his diabetic therapy. You sit down with him and talk about his regimen. He reveals that due to his night job, it is difficult to follow the plan for a.m. and p.m. insulin; so he usually skips it. Together you work on a plan of care that will fit his schedule.

Nurse Researcher: Crossword Puzzle

Across

2. Unknown factors which can cause research findings to be inaccurate
4. Knowledge which is accepted as truth based on expertise
7. Knowledge gained as the result of research
8. The variable which is measured in a research study
9. The process of limiting influencing factors on the dependent variable

Down

1. Knowledge which is passed down from generation to generation
3. Factual material collected during a research study
5. Factors which influence or interfere with results of a study
6. Experimentation aimed at uncovering or collecting facts
7. Careful examination, experimentation or observation of a subject

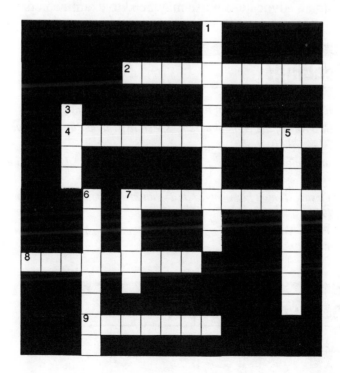

Advocate Role: Short Answer

10. You are caring for Mr. Patrick, who is ready to be discharged home. He has had surgery for colon cancer and has a colostomy. He has received teaching on colostomy care, but is asking you many questions about the basics of caring for his colostomy. He adds that his wife is not willing to help him, or even look at it. As a patient advocate, write down some things you can do for Mr. Patrick to ensure that he and his wife receive follow-up care.

____

____

____

____

____

Advocacy: True/ False

Mark each of the following statements as either TRUE (T) or FALSE (F).

11. ____ All persons need an advocate at some time in their life.
12. ____ Assertive behavior tends to manipulate and dominate other people.
13. ____ Medical records are not available to clients.
14. ____ Nursing places much importance on client's rights.
15. ____ Clients do not always have the right to make their own decision.
16. ____ Advocacy does not involve ethical decisions.
17. ____ Before being an advocate, a nurse may need to examine personal attitudes and values.

Suggested Readings

Clark L, Quinn J: The new entrepreneurs. Nursing and Health Care 9(1):6-15, 1988

Dubrey RJ: The leadership role of the clinical nursing specialists: a quality of life nursing model. Nursing Management 19(5):71-4, 78,80, 1988

Fine RB: Consumerism and information: power and confusion. Nursing Administration Quarterly 12(3):66-73, 1988

Nelson ML: Advocacy nursing: how it has evolved and what are its implcations for practice? Nursing Outlook 36(3):136-41, 1988

Roncoli M, Brooten D, Perez-Woods R: Nursing research: What it costs and who will pay. Nursing and Health Care 9(2):76-80, 1988

Computer Assisted Instruction

Nursing Research. Mosbysystems.

Unit VI
Actions Basic to Nursing Practice

Unit VI focuses on the actions which nurses perform in structured and unstructured settings with clients of all ages, at any point on the health illness continuum. Nursing assessment, meeting safety and security needs, asepsis, and admitting, discharge and home care planning are the focus of this unit.

Chapter 23
Vital Signs

Assessing vital signs, the client's temperature, pulse, respiration, and blood pressure, are considered essential elements in evaluating the client's health status. Vital sign assessment is a part of most agency's admission procedures. Chapter 23 of Fundamentals of Nursing (Taylor, 1988) provides opportunity for the learner to gain knowledge of the relationships between vital signs and body functioning and the procedures for obtaining accurate vital sign assessments.

After studying this chapter and completing the workbook exercises, the learner should be able to

- Define key terms used in the chapter.
- Define the phrase *vital signs.*
- Discuss nursing responsibilities in assessing temperature, pulse, respirations, and blood pressure.
- Compare normal and abnormal vital sign assessments including causes, effects, and implications of abnormal findings.
- Describe the equipment necessary to assess vital signs.
- Identify sites for assessing temperature, pulse and blood pressure.

Key Terms Chapter 23

Prior to attempting the workbook exercises for Chapter 23 it is advisable to become familiar with the key terms used in the chapter.

adventitious sounds
antipyretic
apical-radial pulse rate
apnea
arrhythmia
auscultation
blood pressure
bigeminal pulse
biot's respirations
bradycardia
bradypnea
cardiac output
cardinal signs
Cheyne-Stokes respirations
circadian rhythm
conduction
constant fever
convection
core temperature
crisis
diastolic pressure
dyspnea
dysrhythmia
essential hypertension
eupnea
evaporation
exhalation
expiration
external respiration
fever
friction rub
homeothermic
hyperpyrexia
hypertension
hypotension
hypothermia
inhalation
inspiration
intermittent fever
intermittent pulse
internal respiration
Korotkoff sounds
lysis
meniscus
orthopnea
orthostatic hypotension
palpitation
parallax
peripheral resistance
poikilothermic
polypnea
postural hypotension
premature beat
primary hypertension
pulse
pulse deficit
pulse pressure
pyrexia
radiation
rales
relapsing fever
remittent fever
respiration
rhonchi
secondary hypertension
set point
sinoatrial node
sphygmomanometer
stertorous breathing
stridor
stroke volume
systolic pressure
tachycardia
tachypnea
temperature
tissue respiration
vital signs
wheeze

Vital Signs: Match

Directions: Match the term with the definition.

Terms:

A. apnea
B. arrhythmia
C. bradycardia
D. eupnea
E. dyspnea
F. hyperpyrexia
G. Korotkoff sounds
H. orthopnea
I. stridor
J. tachycardia
K. hypothermia

Definitions:

1. ____ Difficult or labored respirations
2. ____ Rapid respirations above 30 per minute a for an adult
3. ____ Slow heart beat below 60 per a minute in an adult
4. ____ A body temperature below the lower limits of normal
5. ____ Normal respiration
6. ____ A high temperature above 41C
7. ____ Absence of respiration
8. ____ An irregular pattern of heart beat
9. ____ A harsh high pitched sound heard on inspiration, often seen in children with croup
10. ____ A series of sounds heard when measuring arterial blood pressure

Vital Sign: Paragraph Definitions

Read the following nursing situation. Define each of the italicized terms below:

Mary Jones, R.N., was beginning her morning assessment rounds with her clients. She picked up her *sphygmomanometer* and entered the first client's room. She greeted him and began her assessments with an observation of the client and by taking his *vital signs*. She noted that he was *pyrexic,* had a slightly elevated *pulse rate*, and was *tachypneic.* His *systolic pressure* was 120, but she was concerned about his *diastolic pressure* which was 96. She recorded this data temporarily on her note pad and continued her assessment.

11. sphygmomanometer ____________________
12. vital signs ____________________
13. pyrexic ____________________
14. pulse rate ____________________
15. tachypneic ____________________
16. systolic pressure ____________________
17. diastolic pressure ____________________

Vital Signs: Completion

Fill in the blanks to complete the following sentences.

18. The body temperature of a healthy person is maintained within a fairly constant range by the __________ of the brain.
19. The cycling pattern of environmental and physiologic processes in humans is referred to as __________.
20. A very high fever, usually above 41C (105.8F) is referred to as ___________.
21. The transfer of heat to another object during direct contact is called ___________.
22. Before obtaining a rectal temperature the thermometer must be shaken down and ________.
23. When a person feels weak or faint when rising quickly, he may have _____________ .
24. The procedure of listening for sounds within the body is referred to as _________.
25. The most commonly assessed pulse is the _______ _______.
26. The difference between systolic pressure and diastolic pressure is referred to as _____ ________.
27. An axillary temperature is taken under the ______.

Additional Enrichment Activities

1. Comparison of temperature readings by various methods:
   - A. Take oral and axillary temperatures on five different individuals using glass clinical thermometers.
   - B. Take oral and axillary temperatures using electronic thermometers. Chart your assessments in the table below and compare. Explain the findings obtained.

METHOD			
GLASS ORAL	GLASS AXILLARY	ELECTRONIC ORAL	ELECTRONIC AXILLARY
1.			
2.			
3.			
4.			
5.			

Explanation of differences:

____

____

2. Comparison of blood pressure readings by client position:
Take blood pressures on five individuals in lying, sitting, and standing positions. Chart your findings below and explain the similarities and/or differences in the readings.

POSITION			
Person	**Lying**	**Sitting**	**Standing**
1.			
2.			
3.			
4.			
5.			

Explanation of differences:

____

____

3. Check with your local health department and find when they are having their next blood pressure clinic. Participate in the clinic and note the diversity of blood pressures. What are people with hypertension doing to lower their blood pressure levels?

4. Case Study: Mrs. Jane Doe, a 45 year old woman, is a patient on your unit. She was admitted with abdominal pain resulting in a cholecystectomy. Her convalescence was uneventful. While in the hospital, it was discovered that she was hypertensive, and is a borderline diabetic. Mrs. Doe is 5'4", and weighs 232 lbs. She is on a low calorie and low salt diet. Mrs. Doe is outgoing and highly motivated. Her vital signs are normal except for her blood pressure, which ranges from 160/105 to 200/118. Prepare a nursing care plan with Mrs. Doe. Be creative and brief.
   A. Assess her situation.
   B. Prepare a list of potential or relevant nursing diagnoses.

C. Establish nursing care goals.
D. List nursing actions to achieve the established goals.
E. Discuss how the plan will be implemented.
F. Discuss evaluation techniques to be uesd.

Suggested Readings

Becker KL Et Al: Get in touch and tune with cardiac assessment. Nursing 18(3): 51-55, 1988

Bressack, MA Et Al: Importance of venous return, venous resistance, and mean circulatory pressure in the physiology and management of shock. Chest 92(5): 906-912, 1987

Dodman N: Newborn temperature control. Neonatal Network 5(6): 19-23, 1987

Green M: Hypothermia: The chiller that may be missed? . . . low body temperature can be triggered by a variety of factors. Geriatric Nursing Home Care 7(12): 20-21, 1987

Hahn K: Think twice about borderline hypertension. Nursing 18(4): 90-91, 1988

Kilmon CA: Home management of children's fevers. J Pediatric Nursing 2(6): 400-404, 1987

Kispert CP: Clinical measurements to assess cardiopulmonary function. Physical Therapy 67(12): 1886-1890, December 1987

Lohmann M: Fever: Different types, different causes. Nursing 18(4): 98-101, 1988

MacDonald MB Et Al: Lifestyle behaviors in treated hypertensive as prediction of blood pressure control. Rehabilitation Nursing 13(2): 82-84, 1988

Memmer MK: Acute orthostatic hypotension. Heart Lung 17(2): 134-143, 1988

Miracle VA: Get in touch and tune with cardiac assessment. Nursing 18(4): 41-47, 1988

O'Brien EL: Clinical thermometry: In need of nursing research. J Pediatric Nursing 3(3): 207-208, 1988

Openbrier DR Et Al: Home oxygen therapy: Evaluation and prescription. American J Nursing 88(2): 192-197, 1988

Taking accurate blood pressure readings. Nursing 18(4): 32J, 32N, April 1988

VanAmeringen MR Et Al: Intrinsic job stress and diastolic blood pressure among female hospital workers. J Occupational Medicine 30(2): 93-97, 1988

York K: The lung and fluid-electrolyte and acid-base imbalances. Nursing Clinics of North Am 22(4): 805-814, 1987

Computer Assisted Instruction

Vital Signs and Physical Assessment. Mosby Systems

Measuring Blood Pressure by the Indirect Method. American Journal of Nursing Educational Services

Skills Simulations. J.B. Lippincott Company

A Software Guide to Physical Examination, J.B. Lippincott Company

Chapter 24
Nursing Assessment

Assessment, the first phase of the nursing process is presented as an integral component of holistic health care. The health history and nursing examination are the focus of the Chapter 24 Fundamentals of Nursing (Taylor, 1988) which concludes with a sample health history to guide the learner.
After studying the chapter and completing the accompanying workbook exercises the learner should be able to

- Define key terms used in the chapter.
- Identify the purposes of the nursing assessment.
- Describe the techniques used during a nursing examination.
- Discuss the importance of client preparation for a nursing assessment.
- Identify equipment used in performing a nursing assessment.
- Describe positioning used for each body system examination.
- Conduct a nursing assessment of each body system in a systematic manner, identifying normal and abnormal findings.
- Document significant findings in a concise, descriptive manner.

Key Terms Chapter 24

Prior to begining the workbook exercises the learner will want to become familiar with the following terms used in the chapter.

accommodation
adventitious breath sounds
apnea
asymmetry
auscultation
bilateral
bounding pulse
bruits
bronchovesicular
clubbing
cyanosis
dorsal recumbent position
dullness
ecchymosis
erect position
flatness
flushing
heaves
hyperperistalsis
hyperresonance
inspection
jaundice
knee-chest position
lifts
lithotomy position
nasal speculum
neurologic hammer
ophthalmoscope
otoscope
pallor
palpation
percussion
percussion hammer
periorbital edema
peristalsis
petechiae
pleural friction rub
polyps
precordium
prone position
position
rales
rash
resonance
rhonchi
scar
Sims position
stethoscope
striae
supine position
symmetry
thrills
tremor
tuning fork
turgor
tympany
vaginal speculum
vesicular breathing
wound

Key Terms Match

Match the terms to the definitions.

Terms:

A. accommodation
B. adventitious breath sounds
C. pleural friction rush
D. bruits
E. ecchymosis
F. palpation
G. otoscope
H. murmur
I. resonance
J. rhonchi
K. striae
L. turgor
M. tympany
N. petechiae

Definitions:

1.____ A moderate to loud low pitched sound, percussed over the lung
2.____ A loud drumlike sound heard when percussing the stomach or an air filled organ

3.____ Fullness or elasticity of the skin
4.____ Pupil constricts when looking at a near object and dilates when looking at a distant object
5.____ Breath sounds not normally heard in the lung
6.____ Examination of tissue by feeling
7.____ Sound similar to murmurs heard of major blood vessels
8.____ A collection of blood in subcutaneous tissue causing a purplish color
9.____ Coarse gurgling sounds in the bronchial tube, best heard on expiration
10.____ Fine white of silvery lines caused by stretching
11.____ A grating sound caused by an inflamed pleura rubbing against the chest wall
12.____ Extra heart sounds caused by some disruption of blood flow through the heart
13.____ Instrument used to examine the ear
14.____ Small hemorrhage spots caused by capillary hemorrhage

Positioning for Physical Examination

A variety of positions are utilized during a nursing assessment. Define each of the following positions and draw a line figure to illustrate.

15. Supine	16. Dorsal Recumbent
17. Prone	18. Lithotomy
19. Knee Chest	20. Sims

Cranial Nerve Assessment

List the twelve cranial nerves. Identify as to sensory or motor and explain the function of each.

CRANIAL NERVE	SENSORY/MOTOR	FUNCTION
21. I		
22. II		
23. III		
24. IV		
25. V		
26. VI		
27. VII		
28. VIII		
29. IX		
30. X		
31. XI		
32. XII		

Physical Assessment Recording

Having completed a physical assessment on a client/classmate/family member, record your findings. Use the guide provided in Fundamentals of Nursing (Taylor, 1988:479) for documentation of health history and physical assessment. Use correct terminology.

Additional Enrichment Activities

1. Locate a nurse clinician in your area and interview her as to her responsibilities. Identify areas that are expanded role functions.

Suggested Readings

Bates A: A guide to physical examination and history taking. JB Lippincott Company 1987

Becker KL Et AL: Performing in-depth abdominal assessment. Nursing 18(6): 59-63, June 1988

Jordan, KS: Assessment of the person with acquired immunodeficiency syndrome in the emergency department. J Emergency Nursing 13(6): 342-345, November-December 1987

Lexford WM Et Al: Otoscope update. Patient Care 21(14): 85-87, 90, 92, September 1987

Lierman J: Preoperative assessments: Can we afford to do without them? AORN J 47(2): 586, 588, 590, February 1988

McConnell EA: Getting the feel of lymph node assessment. Nursing 18(8): 54-57, August 1988

Parrino TA: The art and science of percussion. Hospital Practice 22(9): 25-28, September 1987

Poyss AS: Assessment and nursing diagnosis in fluid and electrolyte disorders. Nursing Clinics of N. America 22(4): 773-783, December 1987

Rudolph, A Et Al: The breast physical examination: Its value in early cancer detection. Cancer Nursing 10(2): 100-106, April 1987

Smith CE: Assessing bowel sounds: More than just listening. Nursing 18(2): 42-43, February 1988

Stark JL: A quick guide to urinary tract assessment. Nursing 18(7): 54-57, July 1988

Steele, SM: Assessing developmental delays in preschool children. J Pediatric Health Care 2(3): 141-145, May-June 1988

Stevens S Et Al: How to perform picture-perfect respiratory assessment. Nursing 18(1): 57-63, January 1988

Yacone LA: Cardiac assessment: What to do, how to do it. RN 50(5): 42-48, May 1987

Computer Assisted Instruction

A Software Guide to Physical Examination. JB Lippicott

Neurological Nursing: The Neurological Assessment, Medi-Sim

Chapter 25
Safety and Asepsis

The basic human needs of safety and security form the basis for Chapter 25 of Fundamentals of Nursing (Taylor, 1988). Environmental safety in the home and in health care agencies, infection control and prevention, and isolation and communicable disease are the primary topics.

After studying this chapter and completing the workbook exercises, the learner should be able to

- Define key terms used in the chapter.
- Identify factors that may be safety hazards in the client's environment.
- Describe ways in which the client's safety can be promoted in the home and health-care setting.
- Identify clients at risk of falling.
- Describe preventive strategies to decrease the incidence of client falls.
- Identify nursing diagnoses associated with a client in an unsafe situation.
- Describe nursing responsibilities for fire safety.
- Explain the infection cycle.
- Describe nursing interventions used to break the chain of infection.
- List the stages of an infection.
- Identify clients at risk of developing an infection.
- Identify factors that reduce the incidence of nosocomial infection.
- Identify situations in which handwashing is indicated.
- Identify nursing diagnoses associated with a client who has an infection or is at risk of developing an infection.
- Identify protocols for each isolation category.
- Describe recommended techniques for medical and surgical asepsis.

Key Terms Chapter 25

The learner will find it helpful to become familiar with the key terms used in Chapter 25 prior to attempting the workbook exercises.

antigen
antibody
asepsis
medical asepsis
surgical asepsis
carrier
Centers for Disease Control
colonize
convalescent period
disinfectant
disinfection
endogenous
exit from the reservoir
exogenous
fomite
full stage of illness
ground
host
iatrogenic infection
immune response
incident report
incubation period
infection
inflammatory response
isolation
localized symptoms
macroshock
microshock
normal flora
nosocomial infection
pathogen
portal of entry
prodromal stage
reservoir
resident bacteria or flora
restraint
sterilization
suffocation
susceptibility
systemic symptoms
transient bacteria or flora
vector
vehicle
virulence

Key Terms

Match the terms to the definitions.

Terms:

A. asepsis
B. carrier
C. disinfectant
D. fomites
E. iatrogenic
F. pathogen
G. prodromal stage
H. reservoir
I. pandemic
J. vector
K. vehicle
L. virulence

Definitions

1. ____ An infection that occurs as a result of treatment or diagnostic test
2. ____ Individual that has the organism, but not the symptoms of a disease
3. ____ Any activity that prevents infection or breaks the chain of infection
4. ____ Contaminated food, water or inanimate object
5. ____ The most infectious period of the infection stage
6. ____ A substance that destroys pathogenic organisms except spores

7. ____ Any microorganism capable of causing disease
8. ____ Natural habitat for microorganism
9. ____ Excess disease spreading and occurring in man
10. ____ The strength of an organism or its ability to cause disease
11. ____ The means of transmitting organism from one place to another
12. ____ A mosquitoe which transmits disease

Accident Proofing a Home

Many accidents occur in the home. You are visiting the Jones family as part of your caseload in community health. Mrs. Jones wants help in making her home accident free. The Jones' have three children, ages five, three, and one year old. What would be potential dangers specific to each room? What would you suggest to make each room/area accident free?

13. Kitchen:

____

____

____

14. Living room:

____

____

____

15. Bedrooms:

____

____

____

16. Bathroom:

____

____

____

17. Porch and yard:

____

____

____

Infectious Disease: Table Completion

If the Category-Specific Isolation System is the established protocol for an agency, the client's diagnoses determines the isolation procedures to implement. For the diseases listed below identify the causative organism, method of transmission, and the category of isolation indicated. Be specific as to the need for gown, mask, gloves, and handwashing.

INFECTION CONTROL CATEGORY		
Disease	**Causative Organism**	**Gown/Mask/Glove/Handwashing**
18. Pharyngeal diphtheria		
19. Wound infection		
20. Tuberculosis		
21. Gas gangrene		
22. Burn infection		
23. Meningitis		
24. Hepatitis		
25. Malaria		
26. Typhoid		
27. AIDS		

Additional Enrichment Activities

1. Explore the goals and functions of the Centers for Disease Control, Atlanta, Georgia.
2. Go to the clinical learning laboratory for focused practice in the following:
   A. Putting on sterile gloves
   B. Opening sterile dressing and applying them without breaking technique
   C. Putting on isolation mask and gloves
3. Have a classmate apply wrist and waist restraints to you while you are in a hospital bed. Become aware of how it feels to be restrained, and how much activity is permitted by the restraints. How long can you tolerate the restraint? Have a waist restraint applied while you are sitting in a wheelchair and observe your response to this restraint.
4. Write a brief essay on the legal aspects of physical restraint in the hospital. Include documentation requirements, standards of practice, and communication with client/family members about the necessity of the restraints.

Suggested Readings

Ivey FD, Gerner HM: Adults Do Get Chickenpox. American Journal of Nursing 87(12):1658-59, 1987
Silver M: Using Restraint. American Journal of Nursing 87(11):1414-15, 1987
Loucks A: Chlamydia An Unheralded Epidemic. American Journal of Nursing 87(7):920-22, 1987
White AB: I'm Not Letting You Go. American Journal of Nursing 87(3):312-13, 1987

Computer Assisted Instruction

Infection control, including handwashing, gowning, and gloving technique. Heshi
Infant Safety: Anticipatory Guidance. Medi-Sim
Asepsis: Principles of Nursing Pracatice. Medi-Sim
Communicable Diseases in Children, Medi-Sim

Chapter 26
Admitting, Discharge, and Home Visits

The nurse has a major responsibility for ensuring continuity of comprehensive health care through the establishment of a plan of care to be followed and coordinated as the client moves through the health-care system.

After studying this chapter and completing the workbook exercises, the learner should be able to

- Define key terms used in the chapter.
- Identify differences and similarities between nursing care in the hospital and home.
- Develop possible nursing diagnoses for a client in the hospital and develop it for home situation.
- Perform a discharge assessment on a hospitalized client and family.
- Be aware of constraints relating to reimbursement in the provision of home health care.

Key Terms Chapter 26

Prior to beginning the workbook exercises the learner will want to become famaliar with the following key terms used in the Chapter.

admission
compliance
discharge planning
home health care
intensive level care
intermediate level care
maintenance level care
noncompliance
psychiataric nurse specialist
rehabililtative level care
respite care

Client Admission

You have just been notified that a patient is being admitted to your unit and will arrive with an IV via stretcher. List five things you will need to do to get this client's room ready prior to his arrival.

1. ______________________________
2. ______________________________
3. ______________________________
4. ______________________________
5. ______________________________

Patient Teaching

Based on the METHOD approach, identify and discuss the six critical areas of teaching to be addressed prior to a client's discharge.

6. M__________: The client will know

____

7. E__________: The client will be assured of

____

8. T__________: The client and family will

____

9. H_____ t_____: The client will

____

10. O________ r______: The client will

11. D________: The client will be able to

Home Visit Assessment: Short Answer

12. When making a home visit assessment, what kind of data would be important concerning the financial status of the family?

Discharge Planning

List five essential components of discharge planning.

13.

14.

15.

16.

17.

Additional Enrichment Activities

1. Contact your local community health agency and make arrangements to accompany a nurse on a home visit. Observe what the nurse's role in the home is, what she does, and how the client responds. Discuss with the nurse her preparation activities for the visit and its evaluation.

2. Using the Elements of a Home Visit Assessment at the end of your textbook chapter (Taylor, 1988:546) assess your own home and family. What are your strengths and weaknesses? How would you plan to strengthen the weaker or problematic areas if you were the home nurse visiting your family?

Suggested Readings

Barron, S: Preadmission made easy. AJN 87(12): 1690-1691, 1987

Brewer C Et Al: Should doctors control discharge? . . . the case for . . . the case against. Nursing Times 84(3): 42-43, 1988

Denholm CJ: The adolescent patient at discharge and in the post-hospitalization environment: A review. Maternal Child Nursing 16(2): 95-102, 1987

Giesy J: Teaching discharge management . . . utilizing a simulation game, Home Pursuit. J Pediatric Nursing 2(5):353-354, 1987

Humphrey CJ: The home as a setting for care: Clarifying the boundaries of practice. Nursing Clinics of North Am 23(2): 305-314, 1988

Krake D: Professional nursing practice moves into the hospital admitting office. Nursing Management 19(1): 17, 20, 1988

Monica ED Et Al: Documentation in home care: Skilled observation. Home Healthcare Nurse 6(1): 39-40, 1988

Mudditt H: Home truths. Nursing Times 83(35): 31-33, 1987

Myers MB: Home care nursing: A review from the field. Public Health Nursing 5(2): 65-67, 1988

Tynan C: Home health hazard assessment. J Gerontological Nursing 13(10): 25-28, 1987

Unit VII
Promoting Healthy Physiologic Responses

The ten chapters that comprise Unit VII of the Fundamentals of Nursing text (Taylor, 1988) focus on information and guidelines essential to nursing practice: hygiene, activity and rest, nutrition, elimination, oxygenation, and fluid and electrolyte balance. As with previous chapters, nursing process is the organizing framework for the content. The learner will want to pay particular attention to the section at the end of each chapter entitled Nursing Process in Clinical Practice.

Chapter 27
Hygiene

Persons who are ill or who are hospitalized or institutionalized may not be able to be responsible for self-hygiene. Nurses are often in situations where they administer, or administer through others, e.g., family members or other members of the health team, personal care for clients. The focus of Chapter 27 (Taylor, 1988) is to provide the learner with knowledge of the multiple factors that affect personal hygiene and of nursing measures to promote personal hygiene. After studying this chapter and completing the accompanying workbook exercises, the learner should be able to

- Define the key terms used in the chapter.
- List five functions of the skin, three factors influencing the skin's condition, and four basic principles that guide practices of skin care.
- Identify factors affecting skin condition and personal hygiene.
- Assess the integumentary system and the adequacy of hygiene self-care behaviors using appropriate interview and physical assessment skills.
- Develop nursing diagnoses related to deficient hygiene measures.
- Describe the priorities of scheduled hygienic care, early morning care, morning care, afternoon care, and evening care.
- Demonstrate the back massage, identifying at least four reasons for including the back massage in daily nursing care.
- Demonstrate techniques used when assisting clients with hygiene measures, including those used when administering various types of baths and those used in cleaning each part of the body.
- Describe agents commonly used on the skin and scalp and precautions to observe in their use.
- Plan, implement, and evaluate nursing care for common problems of the skin and mucous membranes.
- Describe a pressure ulcer and common sites of its development, factors that predispose to its development, and it prevention, staging, and treatment.

Key Terms Chapter 27

The learner will find it beneficial to become familiar with the key terms used in the chapter prior to attempting the workbook exercises.

acne
alopecia
caries
cerumen
ceruminal gland
dandruff
dermis
emollient
epidermis
gingiva
gingivitis
halitosis
inner canthus
integument
integumentary system
ischemia
necrosis
nits
outer canthus
pediculicide
pediculosis (lice)
periodontitis
personal hygiene
plaque
podiatrist
pressure ulcer (decubitus ulcer, bedsore)
pyorrhea
reactive hyperemia
sebaceous glands
sebum
shearing force
tartar

The Integument Short Essay

The individuals' developmental stage and health condition influence the skin. For each age group, list factors that affect skin condition.

1. Infant: ______
2. Child: ______
3. Adolescent: ______
4. Older individual: ______

5. What is the underlying rationale for a towel bath?

______
______
______

6. Explain the procedure for a towel bath.

______
______
______
______
______
______
______
______

7. Explain the reason for antiembolism stockings

8. Explain the procedure for applying antiembolism stockings.

9. Explain the cause of and treatment for the following skin problems.
   A. Dry skin:

   B. Acne:

   C. Skin rashes:

10. Proper foot care
    A. A diabetic client is especially prone to foot problems. There are certain additional precautions that should be observed and taught to the client with diabetes. List the main points of foot care for the diabetic.

    B. Outline proper foot care techniques.

Key Terms: Match

Match the hygiene term with the appropriate definition.

Terms:

A. acne
B. alopecia
C. caries
D. cerumen
E. dermis
F. emollient
G. gingivitis
H. halitosis
I. ischemia
J. necrosis
K. pediculosis
L. podiatrist
M. pyorrhea
N. sebum

Definitions:

11. ___ True layer of skin consists of mooth muscular tissue, nerve, and hair follicles
12 ___ Waxlike soft brown secretion found in the outer ear
13. ___ Offensive breath
14. ___ An inflammatory disease of the sebaceous gland and hair follicles of the skin
15. ___ Decay of teeth
16. ___ An agent that will soften the part when applied locally
17. ___ Inflammation of the gums
18. ___ Absence or loss of hair, usually the head
19. ___ Local deficiency of blood supply due to obstruction of the circulation to a part
20. ___ A fatty secretion of the sebaceous glands of the skin
21. ___ A periodontal disease characterized by inflammation or degenerative changes of the periosteum, alveolar bone, and tooth cementum
22. ___ Death of areas of tissue due to insufficient blood supply
23. ___ Infestation with lice
24. ___ A health professional responsible for the care of the human foot

Additional Enrichment Activities

1. Spend a day in a community health agency. Make a home visit with one of the nurses. What problems are encountered in the home? How does the nurse solve the problems?

2. Mr. Jasper is a 58 year old man admitted to the hospital with rheumatoid arthritis. Mr. Jasper lives alone and has problems with personal hygiene. Mr. Jasper lives in a first floor apartment, and has no family, but he does have several friends that are eager to be helpful. Mr. Jasper has a wheelchair to get around the apartment. You are the community health nurse who will visit Mr. Jasper.
   A. Assess the home situation
   B. Establish nursing diagnoses
   C. Devise a plan of care
   D. Implement the plan
   E. Establish methods to use for evaluation of the plan

Suggested Readings

Bryant RA: Saving the skin from tape injuries. American J Nursing 88(2):189-191, 1988

Byass R: Soothing body and soul...massage. Nursing Times 84(24):39-41, 1988

Harrison A: Oral hygiene: denture care. Nursing Times 83(19):28-29, 1987

Jackson BS et al: The effects of the Clinitron bed on pressure ulcers. J Nursing Administration 17(11):5, 1987

McCord F et al: Brushing up on oral care. Nursing Times 84(13):40-41, 1988

Miller R et al: Oral health care for hospitalized patients: the nurses's role. J Nursing Education 26(9):362-366, 1987

Morris L et al: Nursing the patient in traction. RN 5(1):26-31, 1988

Nicol NH: Atopic Dermatitis: The (Wet) Wrap-Up. American J Nursing (12):1560-63, 1987

Overton E: Bedmaking and bacteria. Nursing Times 84(9):69, 71, 1988

Parrott TE: Care of long hair. AD Nurse 2(5):8-10, 1987

Pritchard V: Geriatric infections: skin and soft tissue. RN 51(6):60-63, 1988

Wienke VK: Pressure sores: prevention is the challenge. Orthopedic Nursing 6(4):26-30, 1987

White JA: Touching with intent: therapeutic massage. Holistic Nursing Practice 2(3):63-67, 1988

Chapter 28
Activity

Your textbook points out that the ability to move is closely related to the fulfillment of other basic human needs. And, for the majority of healthy persons, movement is taken for granted. Chapter 28, Fundamentals of Nursing (Taylor, 1988) provides the student with knowledge of the physiology of movement, the principles of body mechanics, and factors affecting body alignment and mobility. The nursing process provides the organizing theme for this content.

After studying this chapter and completing the workbook exercises the learner should be able to

- Define key terms used in this chapter.
- Describe the role of the skeletal, muscular, and nervous systems in the physiology of movement.
- Identify seven variables that influence body alignment and mobility.
- Differentiate isotonic, isometric, and isokinetic exercise.
- Describe the effects of exercise and immobility on major body systems.
- Assess body alignment, mobility, and activity tolerance, utilizing appropriate interview questions and physical assessment skills.
- Develop nursing diagnoses that correctly identify mobility problems amenable to nursing therapy.
- Utilize proper body mechanics when positioning, moving, lifting, and ambulating clients.
- Design exercise programs.
- Plan, implement, and evaluate nursing care related to select nursing diagnoses involving mobility problems.

Key Terms Chapter 28

The learner is advised to become familiar with the Key Terms used in Chapter 28 prior to attempting the workbook exercises.

abduction
active exercise
active-assistive exercise
adduction
aerobic exercise
ankylosis
atelectasis
atrophy
base of support
body mechanics
center of gravity
contractures
dangling
disuse osteoporosis
dorsiflexion
endurance
eversion
extension
external rotation
fitness
flaccidity
flexibility
flexion
footdrop
Fowler's position
hemiplegia
hyperextension
internal rotation
inversion
isokinetic exercise
isometric exercise
isotonic exercise
line of gravity
movement/daily life activities
orthopedics
osteoporosis
paraplegia
passive exercise
plantar flexion
pronation
prone position
range of motion
rotation
semi-Fowler's position
spasticity
strength
strength and endurance exercises
stretching exercises
supination
supine position
Sims' position
synovial joints
tonus
target heart range

Body Position and Movements: Match

Match the terms with the appropriate definitions

Terms:

A. body mechanics
B. center of gravity
C. line of gravity
D. base of support
E. strength and endurance exercises
F. movement/activities
G. atelectasis
H. hemiplegia
I. foot-drop
J. active-assistive exercises
K. abduction
L. adduction
M. disuse osteoporosis
N. dorsiflexion
O. eversion
P. extension
Q. external rotation
R. flexion
S. hyperextension
T. internal rotation
U. inversion
V. plantar flexion
W. rotation
X. supination

Definitions:

1. ____ Exercise that will increase the power of the musculoskeletal system and generally improve the whole body
2. ____ A vertical line that passes through the center of gravity
3. ____ A second person provides minimal support while the client does exercise
4. ____ An incomplete expansion or collapse of lung tissue
5. ____ The foot is unable to maintain itself in the perpendicular position
6. ____ Housecleaning, climbing stairs, caring for others, etc.
7. ____ The point at which a mass is centered
8. ____ Paralysis of one-half of the body
9. ____ The foundation that provides for an object's stability
10. ____ The efficient use of the body as a machine and as a means of locomotion
11. ____ Bone formation slows with a net loss of calcium, phosphorus and matrix
12. ____ Lateral movement of a body part away from the midline
13. ____ The assumption of the supine position
14. ____ Movement of the sole of the foot outward
15. ____ Turning of a body part on the axis provided by its joint
16. ____ Movement of the sole of the foot inward
17. ____ Lateral movement of a body part toward the midline
18. ____ The state of exaggerated extension
19. ____ Backward bending of the hand or foot
20. ____ Flexion of the foot
21. ____ A body part turning on its axis toward the midline
22. ____ The state of being in a straight line
23. ____ The state of being bent
24. ____ A body part turning on its axis away from the midline

Crossword puzzle

Across

3. independent movement of joints through full range of motion
5. paralysis of the legs
6. permanent shortening of muscles
8. freely moveable joints in which there is a space between the articulating bones
12. the term used to describe the state of slight contraction in which we normally find skeletal muscles
14. exercise that involves muscle shortening and actual movement
15. muscles that have decreased tone or hypotonicity
16. activities of daily living
17. exercise involving muscle contraction without shortening
19. exercises that allow muscles and joints to be moved gently through their full range of motion to crease flexibility
21. exercises involving muscle contractions with resistance

Down

1. bone demineralization
2. semi-sitting position with head elevated 45-60 degrees
3. decreased muscle size
4. position of lying on the side with lower arm behind and upper arm flexed at both the shoulder and elbow
7. muscles with increased tone that interferes with movement and caused by neurological impairment
9. the correction or prevention of disorders of the boy's structures for locomotion
10. consolidation and immobilization of a joint
11. exercise where a second person moves joints through range of motion
13. head-of-bed range of motion
15. exercise with sustained muscle movements that increase blood flow, heart rate, and metabolic for oxygen
18. complete extent of movement of which a joint is normally capable
20. to sit on the edge of the bed with legs and feet over the side

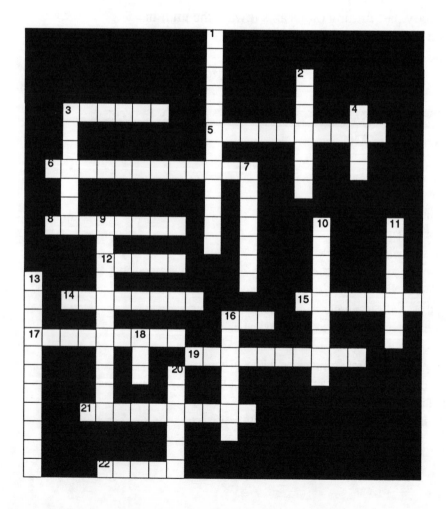

Body Mechanics: Short Answer

Answer the following questions in the space provided

25. Name seven factors that affect body alignment and mobility.
    A. ______
    B. ______
    C. ______
    D. ______
    E. ______
    F. ______
    G. ______
26. List eight good body mechanic guidelines.
    A. ______
    B. ______
    C. ______
    D. ______
    E. ______
    F. ______
    G. ______
    H. ______
27. Describe four things a nurse who is an effective role model for healthy mobility behaviors would do.
    A. ______
    B. ______
    C. ______
    D. ______
28. What does physical assessment of mobility include?

______
______
______
______
______
______
______

29. List the basic guidelines for the nurse when helping to put the client's joints through range of motion.

______
______
______
______

30. What guidelines should nurses follow when moving and lifting clients?

31. What are quadriceps drills? When would you use them?

32. List the criteria for ambulating a client?

33. You are given the order to measure and obtain axillary crutches for your client. How do you do this? What are some ways to help your client prepare for crutch walking?

34. Describe the four crutch gaits and when you would use them.

A.

B.

C.

D.

35. What is involved in the process of exercise prescription for a client?

36. The art of positioning makes sense when you base everything you do on preparing your client for the day when bed rest is no longer required. What do you do to maintain a good body alignment when positioning a client on their side?

Case Study

Bill, age 60, is admitted with pain in his right knee on movement that is relieved by rest. There is a history of trauma to this knee. Physical assessment reveals local tenderness with no redness or warmth; limited motion due to pain; muscle wasting; and obesity.

37. Identify at least three nursing diagnoses.

    A. ______________________________

    ____

    B. ______________________________

    ____

    C. ______________________________

    ____

Additional Enrichment Activities

1. Measure one of your peers for crutches. Borrow the correct size from the physical therapy department and become familiar with the different gaits.
2. Determine the most common contracture seen in the unconscious or immobilized client. Practice positions and make devices that could be useful, ie. handrolls out of available linen, etc.
3. Certain aspects must be documented in the client's record every shift or every twenty-four hours to comply with quality assurance. Identify those aspects that involve your client's mobility status of skin condition.
4. The normal aging process has its implications for nursing practice. Determine physical changes that will occur that may affect a client's mobility and write a care plan.
5. Draw a picture and write a descriptin of each of the following types of joints.

a. ball and socket	d. hinge
b. pivote	e. saddle
c. glidinge	f. condyloid

Suggested Readings

Holmes R, et al: Nutrition Know-How Combating Pressure Sores-Nutritionally. American J Nursing 87(10):1301-03, 1987

Providing early mobility. Nursing Photobook. Horsham, PA, Intermed Communications, 1980

Rubin M: The Physiology of Bed Rest. American J Nursing 88(1):50-55, 1988

Chapter 29
Rest and Sleep

In Chapter 29 of the Fundamentals of Nursing text (Taylor,1988), the learner is given opportunity to gain knowledge of the functions and physiology of sleep, dreams and dream theories, and factors affecting sleep. Nursing diagnoses related to the sleep disturbances of insomnia and sleep deprivation are presented in case study format.

After studying this chapter and completing the workbook exercises, the learner should be able to

- Define key terms used in this chapter.
- Describe the functions and physiology of sleep.
- Identify 11 variables that influence rest and sleep.
- Describe nursing implications for age-related differences in the sleep-wakefulness cycle.
- Perform a comprehensive sleep assessment using appropriate interview questions, a sleep diary when indicated, and physical assessment skills.
- Describe common sleep disorders noting key assessment criteria.
- Develop nursing diagnoses that correctly identify sleep problems that may be treated by independent nursing intervention.
- Describe nine nursing strategies to promote rest and sleep, and identify their rationale.
- Plan, implement, and evaluate nursing care related to select nursing diagnoses involving sleep problems.

Key Terms Chapter 29

circadian rhythm
circadian synchronization
delta sleep
electroencephalograph (EEG)
electromyogram (EMG)
electrooculogram (EOG)
enuresis
hypersomnia
insomnia
narcolepsy
nocturnal myoclonus
nonrapid eye movement (NREM)
parasomnias
rapid eye movement (REM)
rest
sleep
sleep apnea
sleep cycle
sleep deprivation
somnambulism

Key Terms Match

Match the terms or phrases with their corresponding definitions. Place the number of the term or phrase in the blank at the left of the definition.

Terms:

a. arousal threshold
b. circadian rhythm
c. circadian synchronization
d. delta sleep
e. electroencephalograph (EEG)
f. electromyogram (EMG)
g. electrooculogram (EOG)
h. enuresis
i. hypersomnia
j. insomnia
k. narcolepsy
l. nocturnal myoclonus
m. NREM
n. parasomnias
o. REM
p. rest
q. sleep
r. sleep apnea
s. sleep cycle
t. sleep deprivation
u. somnambulism

Definitions:

1. ____ Bedwetting during sleep
2. ____ Designates a stage of sleep characterized by autonomic activation, muscle paralysis, and characteristic eye movements
3. ____ A state achieved when the body's inner clocks operate in harmony with each other, results in feelings of well being
4. ____ Difficulty initiating or maintaining sleep
5. ____ Sleepwalking
6. ____ Graphic record of eye movements
7. ____ State of sleep characterized by slow wave, high voltage brain electrical activity

8. ____ Group of disorders characterized by troublesome activities occurring during sleep, mainly Stage IV
9. ____ State of altered consciousness characterized by body inactivity and cycles of brain activity
10. ____ The point at which external stimulus will awaken the sleeper
11. ____ Graphic record of electrical activity produced by muscle contraction
12. ____ A condition produced by too little sleep or blockage of any stage of sleep
13. ____ That portion of sleep stages characterized by muscle relaxation and lowered measure of blood pressure, respiratory rate, pulse and temperature
14. ____ Period of 90-100 minutes during sleep when brain activity moves from Stage I to Stage IV sleep and back again to Stage I REM sleep
15. ____ Twenty four hour fluctuation in body activity, organ function, hormone secretion and metabolism
16. ____ Sleep disorder characterized by uncontrollable desire to sleep and sleep onset REM sleep
17. ____ Sleep disorder characterized by long periods of not breathing, resulting in anoxia
18. ____ State characterized by inactivity and subsequent subjective refreshment
19. ____ State characterized by sleep for excessive periods of time
20. ____ Graphic record of electrical activity occurring within the brain
21. ____ Sleep disorder characterized by rhythmic muscle contractions (particularly of the leg and foot) during sleep

Case Study

22. Read the following case study, answer the questions and fill in the blanks.

Steve Erickson, age 55, comes into the health clinic complaining of feeling extremely fatigued; in fact, he has had to give up one of his main pleasures, golf. He is an accountant and reports that his boss is "on his back" all the time. He blames his problems with his job on his fatigue; in fact, he has a hard time staying awake at work. His wife, Geneva, reports that she is becoming extremely frustrated with their marriage. Steve is irritable and "snaps at me" all the time. She complains that he will not go anywhere anymore, but sits in front of the television every evening and falls asleep. He then just gets up and goes on to bed. He snores so loud she has trouble sleeping. Steve is five foot ten inches tall, and weights 250 pounds. His blood pressure is elevated and lately he complains of mild chest pain upon exertion.

A. What additional information do you need to complete your assessment?

____

____

____

____

B. List nursing diagnoses obtained from your data:

____

____

C. List goals for Steve.

D. List goals for Geneva.

Steve has been referred to a sleep disorder clinic for evaluation. He was diagnosed with sleep apnea. His physician gave him instructions to lose fifty pounds and to stay off his back during sleep.

E. What is the rationale for this?

F. Was one of your nursing diagnoses: Sleep Pattern Disturbance, Excessive daytime sleepiness related to disturbed nocturnal sleep secondary to sleep apnea? _______

G. For this diagnosis, write one appropriate nursing goal for Steve.

H. You goal should direct your plan of care for Steve. What nursing activities can you initiate to help Steve function better in the daytime?

I. Steve and Geneva need a lot of information about sleep apnea, the problems it has been causing in their lives and steps they can take to improve Steve's sleep, his function and their relationship. What will you teach Steve? Geneva? (Hint - You may need to look up sleep apnea in a nursing journal to help you)

J. After you have done all the above, how will you know if what you did achieved the goal you established?

23. Plan an instruction sheet to use for general guidelines for planning care for all adult patients to enhance their sleep on a hospital nursing unit.
    A. What guidelines will there be for providing an environment conducive to sleep?
    B. How will these guidelines be altered for an elderly person?
    C. What do you want to include about work activities while working the night shift?
    D. Do you want to include something about how you will organize your nursing care?
    E. What time of day will you plan to encourage your patients to get out of bed and become as active as possible?
    F. What general plans would help you to provide evening activities conducive to sleep?

G. What general health teaching do you plan to include? Will you include any diet suggestions?

____

____

Additional Enrichment Activities

1. Keep a sleep diary on yourself for twenty four hours. (See page 701-704 for more specific guidelines.) Include:
   A. Time you go to bed
   B. Time you began to try to sleep
   C. Time you went to sleep
   D. Time of any nocturnal awakenings
   E. Time you awaken in the morning
   F. Time you actually get out of bed

Also record the following during waking hours:
   A. Any naps taken (record times)
   B. When you ate - record light meals (LM), moderate meals (MM), or heavy meals (HM); snacks (S
   C. Any caffeinated beverages (C)
   D. Any alcoholic beverages (A)
   E. Any medication taken (M)
   F. Periods of physical exercise, light (LE), moderate (ME), or heavy (HE)
   G. What did you learn about your patterns of sleep?
   H. What could you identify about your sleep-activity patterns that were health promoting?
   I. What did you identify about your sleep-activity patterns that detract from your well-being?
2. Interview an elderly person about his/her sleep. Include their perception and their description of their sleep pattern. Also include as much as is possible the data you would record in a sleep lab.
3. Interview a middle-aged person about his/her sleep patterns in the same way that you interviewed the elderly person. What differences did you observe? Were they ones you would expect from the age difference?
4. Interview a young adult about his/her sleep patterns. Compare these sleep patterns with the ones you found previously.
5. Interview a parent of a small child. Ask them to describe a typical twenty four hour sleep pattern for their child. Include activity levels, eating patterns, and such data as nightmares, sleep walking or talking and bedwetting. How did the parent's description compare with your expectations about a child's sleeping and activity patterns?
6. Select a sleeping disorder. Go to the library and find and read an article in a nursing journal on that disorder.
7. Visit a sleep laboratory. Observe several tracings of EEG's. Ask the technologist or the physician to explain the tracings. Can you identify the sleep stages from the tracings? Do the tracings from two different individuals look very similar for the correspnding sleep stage?

Suggested Readings

Alward, RR: Are you a lark or an owl on the night shift? American J of Nursing 88(10):1336-1339, 1988

Class, J: Patients' sleep-wake rhythms in hospital. Nursing Times 84(1):48-50, 1988

Fernsebner, B: Chronobiology and institutional influences on the operating room nurse's level of wellness. Perioperative Nursing Quarterly 3(3):23-33, 1987

Geach, B: Bedtime ceremonial: a focus for nursing...heightened significance in psychiatric settings. Archives of Psychiatric Nursing 1(2):98-103, 1987

Kavey, NB et al: Why every patient needs a good night's sleep. RN 49(12):16-19, 1986

Keefe, MR: The impact of infant rooming-in on maternal sleep at night. J of Obstetric Gynecologic, and Neonatal Nursing 17(2):122-126, 1988

Morgan, K: And so to sleep...sleep in later life. Nursing Times 84(12):40-41, 1988

Oesting, HH et al: Sleep apnea. Geriatric Nursing 9(4):232-233, 1988

Pictorial: Snoring. Hospital Medicine 23(12):101-102,107, 1987

Powell, GM et al: Maternal anxiety and the nature of sleep onset latency in hospitalized children. Pediatric Nursing 13(6):397-400, 1987

Ryan, L et al: Impact of Circadian rhythm research on approaches to affective illness. Archives of Psychiatric Nursing 1(4): 236-240, 1987

Verhagen, P et al: The adaptation of night nurses to different work schedules. Ergonomics 30(9):1301-1309, 1987

Young, SH et al: Managing nocturnal wandering behavior. J Gerontological Nursing 14(5):6-12,38-39, 1988

Chapter 30
Comfort

Study of this chapter of Fundamentals of Nursing (Taylor, 1988) will provide the learner with knowledge of the pain experience and factors that influence it. Specific nursing strategies for promoting comfort and pain management are discussed.
After studying this chapter, the learner should be able to

- Define key terms used in the chapter.
- Describe specific elements in the pain experience.
- Compare and contrast acute and chronic pain.
- Identify factors that may affect an individual's pain experience.
- Obtain a complete pain assessment utilizing appropriate interviewing and physical assessment skills.
- Develop nursing diagnoses that correctly identify pain problems and demonstrate the relationship between pain and other areas of human functioning.
- Demonstrate the correct use of no-invasive pain-relief measures: distraction, relaxation, cutaneous stimulation.
- Administer analgesic agents safely to produce the desired level of analgesia without causing undesirable side-effects.
- Collaborate with the members of other health disciplines employing different treatment modalities to promote pain relief.
- Plan, implement, and evaluate nursing care related to select nursing diagnoses for pain problems.
- Utilize teaching and counseling skills to empower clients to direct their own pain management programs.

Key Terms Chapter 30

Prior to attempting the workbook exercises the learner should become familiar with the following key terms used in the text.

acupressure
acupuncture
acute pain
analgesic drug
brief pain
cutaneous stimulation
continuous pain
contralateral stimulation
chronic pain
diffuse pain
dull pain
endorphins
excruciating pain
gate control theory
hypnosis
imagery
ntermittent pain
mild pain
moderate pain
pain
pain threshold
pain tolerance
phantom limb pain
placebo
psychogenic pain
referred pain
relax
severe pain
sharp pain
shifting pain
slight pain
somatic pain
transient pain
visceral pain

Match

Read the following statements and select the term which best describes the client's pain. You may use the term more than once.

Terms:

A. Acute
B. Chronic
C. Intermittent
D. Transient
E. Mild
F. Dull
G. Diffuse
H. Sharp
I. Severe
J. Shifting

Definitions:

1. ____ "Sometimes I think the pain is gone for good, but then it always comes back."
2. ____ "Well, yesterday the pain was up here, but today it seems to be more in this area."
3. ____ "I fractured it yesterday. The pain was so bad I thought I would pass out."
2. ____ "Well, yesterday the pain was up here, but today it seems to be more in this area."
3. ____ "I fractured it yesterday. The pain was so bad I thought I would pass out."
4. ____ "The pain is not constant, but I've had it for over two years now."
5. ____ "Well, it's not exactly sharp or severe, but it is constant and aching."
6. ____ "I can't tell exactly, it feels like my entire body is hurting."
7. ____ "It just lasts a second, but it really does hurt when it's there."
8. ____ "It's an intense, stabbing kind of pain."

9. ____ "My head hurts so bad I can hardly tolerate it."
10. ____ "I guess my tonsils are really swollen and red. They feel just awful. I can hardly swallow."
11. ____ "It wouldn't be so bad, but the pain just never goes away. I've had this for about a year."

Pain Syndromes

Match the following pain syndromes with their defining characteristics.

Pain Syndromes:

A. Causalgia
B. Postherpetic neuralgia
C. Phantom
D. Headache
E. Trigeminal neuralgia
F. Psychogenic
G. Intervertebral disc
H. Arthritis
I. Thalamic
J. Myofascial

Pain Characteristics:

12. ____ dull, aching pain in the muscles and fascia often combined with muscle spasms
13. ____ most common of the deep somatic types of pain
14. ____ burning, diffuse pain occurring in the area of a partially injured peripheral nerve
15. ____ severe, spontaneous pain on the lateral side of a lesion in the thalamus
16. ____ pain along the dorsal root ganglia following a CNS infection with the herpes zoster virus
17. ____ paroxysms of lightning-like intense stabs of pain affecting the mouth, gums, cheek and surface of the head.
18. ____ burning, crushing or cramping pain felt in an amputated limb
19. ____ chronic, painful disease of connective tissue especially common in North America
20. ____ pain associated with a ruptured or herniated intervertebral lower back or cervical disc

Analgesia

Differentiate between the following analgesic medications.

Medication	Action	Major Side Effect	Narcotic (yes/no)
21. Morphine			
22. Demerol			
23. Aspirin			

Patient Goal Statements

Write an appropriate patient goal for each of the following nursing diagnoses.

24. Ineffective individual coping related to family inability to emotionally support client during pain experience.
____
25. Self care deficit related to painful movement of joints.
____
26. Alteration in comfort: left leg pain related to fractured femur and multiple lacerations.
____
27. Alteration in comfort: acute postoperative pain related to fear of taking prescribed analgesia.
____
28. Ineffective airway clearance related to acute post-operative pain.
____

Pain Responses

Label the following responses to pain as:

A. Behavioral *B. Physiological* *C. Affective*

Pain Response:

29. ____ anorexia
30. ____ pupil dilation
31. ____ rapid and irregular breathing
32. ____ hopelessness
33. ____ restlessness
34. ____ moving away from painful stimuli
35. ____ pallor
36. ____ depression
37. ____ anxiety
38. ____ refusal to move
39. ____ fainting
40. ____ increased (or decreased) blood pressure
41. ____ fear
42. ____ moaning, crying
43. ____ nausea and vomiting
44. ____ powerlessness

Key Term Definitions

45. Define the following key terms:
    - A. Analgesia:____________________________
    - B. Diffuse Pain:__________________________
    - C. Pain Tolerance:________________________
    - D. Pain Threshold:________________________
    - E. Psychogenic Pain: ______________________

Crossword Puzzle

Complete the crossword puzzle, using terms found in Chapter 30.

Across

1. an intense and sticking type of pain
2. intense, unrelenting pain
3. ___ stimulation reduces pain on opposite side of source
4. needle pricking at or near pain source
5. imagining something pleasant or happy
6. body wall pain
7. clients can be reluctant to seek _ when in pain
8. morphine like substance produced by the body
9. pain lasting for more than 6 months
10. music as a distraction may help the client to ____and feel less pain
11. a transcutaneous electrical nerve stimulator used for pain control

Down

1. intense pain rated from 8-10 on a 0-10 scale
2. non-intense, diffuse pain
3. pain removed from area in which stimulus originates
4. pressure applied at or near pain source
5. inactive substance given in place of a drug
6. pain lasting less than 6 months
7. altering the state of one's consciousness
8. to enhance client ___ is a nursing goal
9. plans are made to ____the client's discomfort
10. pain of internal organs
11. pain rated between 1 and 3 on a scale of 0 to 10
12. pain from an amputated limb
13. a ___environment can help relax a client
14. an unpleasant sensation present whenever the client says it is

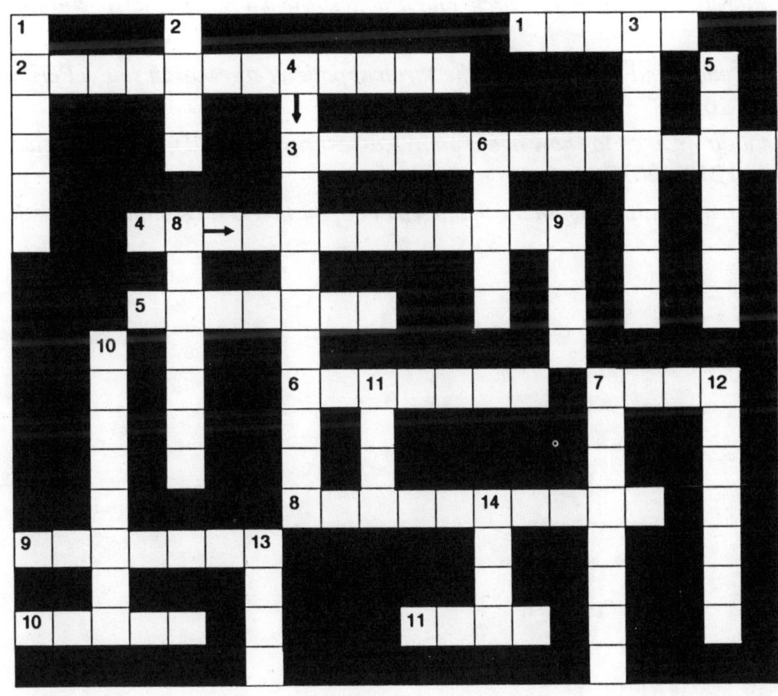

Additional Enrichment Activities

1. In the agency you are assigned to for clinical, examine the methods by which staff assesses and records patient pain status.
2. During one clinical day, list all the examples of different types of pain and pain reactions that you observe.
3. Visit a pain clinic, if there is one in your community, and discuss with the nurses their feelings about pain and its treatment.
4. Recall your last pain experience and note factors that were effective in reducing or controlling your pain. Also note factors that seemed to contribute to your pain.
5. Exchange information with other students regarding their own pain experiences.

Suggested Readings

Beaver, PK: Premature infants' response to touch and pain: can nurses make a difference? Neonatal Network 6(3):13-17, 1987

Behrendt, N: How bad are our kids hurting? a child's perception of pain. Caring 7(6):18-20, 1988

Coyle, N: Analgesics and pain: current concepts. Nursing Clinics of North America 22(3):727-741, 1987

Kleiman, RL et al: PCA vs regular IM injections for severe postop pain. American J Nursing 87(11):1491-1492, 1987

Leckie, RS et al: Uses of acupuncture for pain relief. Hospital Practice 21(12):36i,36o-36p,41, 1986

Lisson, EL: Ethical issues related to pain control. Nursing Clinics of North America 22(3):649-659, 1987

Martinelli, AM: Pain and ethnicity: how people of different cultures experience pain. AORN J 46(2):273-274, 1987

McGuire, DB: Advances in control of cancer pain. Nursing Clinics of North America 22(3):677-690, 1987

Pearson, BD: Pain control: an experiment with imagery. Geriatric Nursing 8(1):28-30, 1987

Perry, SW et al: Pain perception vs pain response in burn patients. American J Nursing 87(5):698, 1987

Stevens, B: Pain in children: theoretical, research, and practice dilemmas. J Pediatric Nursing 2(3):154-166, 1987

Swinford, P: Relaxation and positive imagery for the surgical patient: a research study. Perioperative Nursing Quarterly 3(3):9-16, 1987

Watt-Watson, JH: What do we need to know about pain?...assessing pain and giving narcotics. American J Nursing 87(9):1217-1218, 1987

Wright, SM: The use of therapeutic touch in the management of pain. Nursing Clinics of North America 22(3):705-714, 1987

Chapter 31
Nutrition

Chapter 31 of the Fundamentals of Nursing text (Taylor, 1988) provides the knowledge base of basic nutrition within the framework of two sets of nursing diagnoses. In the first set, the nursing diagnosis is an actual or potential nutritional problem. In the second set of diagnoses explored in the chapter, the nutritional problem is the cause of other diagnoses.

After studying this chapter and completing the workbook exercises the student should be able to

- Define key terms used in the chapter.
- List the six classes of nutrients and explain the significance of each, including variables affecting nutrient requirements.
- Evaluate a diet using the food group approach.
- Identify dietary, medical-socioeconomic, anthropometric, clinical, and biochemical risk factors for poor nutritional status.
- Describe nutritional implications of growth and development throughout the life cycle.
- Perform a nutritional assessment using appropriate interview questions, a 24-hour food recall when indicated, and a nursing examination.
- Describe common nutritional problems noting key assessment criteria.
- Develop nursing diagnoses that correctly identify nutritional problems which may be treated by independent nursing intervention.
- Describe nursing interventions to help clients achieve their nutritional goals.
- Plan, implement, and evaluate nursing care related to selected nursing diagnoses involving nutritional problems.

Key Terms Chapter 31

The learner will want to become familiar with the following key terms prior to attempting the workbook exercises.

amino acid
anorexia
anorexia nervosa
anthropometric
basal metabolism
bulimia
calorie
cholesterol
complete proteins
disaccharides
fatty acid
incomplete proteins
lipid
minerals
monosaccharides
nitrogen balance
nutrition
obesity
overweight
polysaccharides
recommended dietary allowances
specific dynamic action
trace elements
triglycerides
vitamins

Nutrition Terms

Please match the following terms with their appropriate definitions by placing the corresponding definition letter in the space provided in front of the nutrition term.
Nutrition Item:

Definition

A. Substance needed for emulsification of fats
B. Responsible for carrying oxygen from the lungs to the tissues
C. Recommendations for average daily amounts of nutrients to meet nutritional needs
D. Supply energy for the body
E. Introduction of nourishment into the stomach by mechanical means
F. Needed for metabolism of carbohydrates, proteins and fats
G. Amount of energy required for activities of the body at rest
H. Provides the medium for all chemical reactions within the body
I. Contains amounts of all essential amino acids
J. Replacement of body's protein tissues

1. _____ Carbohydrates
2. _____ Vitamins
3. _____ Complete protein
4. _____ Basal metabolism
5. _____ Anabolism
6. _____ Bile
7. _____ RDA
8. _____ Gastric gavage
9. _____ Hemoglobin
10. _____ Water

Nutrition : Completion

Fill in the blanks with the missing word or phrase that would complete the sentence.

11. _______________ provides more than twice the calories per unit than either _______ or ______________ .
12. Another term for Vitamin B_1 is _______________.
13. The __________________ in carrots helps improve visual activity in dim light.
14. Hypokalemia is a less than normal amount of_______________ in the blood.
15. Processed foods, canned meats, pickled foods and foods prepared in brine are all very high in __________________.

Nutrition Crossword Puzzle

Across

2. Unhealthy way to control weight
35. Loss of appetite
76. Protein's basic building blocks
87. Recommended average daily amount of food intake
106. Type of nasogastric tube
112. Energy measured by this
143. 40% of our diet is this (Abrv)
196. Body water outside the cells (Abrv)
203. This is 2/3 of the body's water (Abrv)
213. Obesity theory says there is faulty production of this (Abrv)
232. Body's ideal biological weight

Down

2. Prevents constipation
6. Phosphorous is one of them
27. More vital to life than food
49. Nutrition via a vein
61. Type of vitamin
68. Lactose is an example
108. 9 calories for every gram of this
110. In-depth anthropometric measure (Abrv)
118. Best source of cholesterol
198. Should not be more than 30-35% of total day's calories

2 6 27 35 49 61 68 76 87 106 108 110 112 118 143 196 198 203 213 237

Nutrition Case Study

Mary Brown is 5 feet 2 inches, small framed, and weighs 150 pounds. She has had a weight problem since adolescence. She now is in her thirties and is really motivated to lose weight this time and maintain her weight loss. She is aerobically exercising 30 minutes three times a week.

16. What is Mary's ideal weight? __________.

The Nurse as a Critical Thinker

Nurses have scientific rationale for their nursing interventions. For a change of pace, please provide the intervention that relates to the rationale stated in the following scenario.

The patient, John Black, 65 year old cachectic male, has a nasogastric tube inserted for intermittent feeding purposes. The following interventions occur during the various phases of his hospitalization.

Insertion of the nasogastric tube

19. Rationale - This process facilitates insertion of a rubber NG tube.
    Intervention - ______________________________
20. Rationale - This ensures that the tube will be inserted far enough to enter the stomach.
    Intervention - ______________________________

Feeding Via the NG Tube

21. Rationale - This will confirm the presence of the tube in the stomach.
    Intervention - ______________________________
22. Rationale - Sluggish gastric emptying time will show a residual of 50% of the previous hour's intake.
    Intervention - ______________________________
23. Rationale - This helps the tube feeding enter the stomach by gravity and also decreases the chance of lung aspiration.
    Intervention - ______________________________
24. Rationale - This clears the tube of feeding and prevents blockage of NG tube.
    Intervention - ______________________________

Removing a Nasogastric Tube

25. Rationale - This will allow for easy and unrestricted removal of the tube.
    Intervention - ______________________________
26. Rationale - This will prevent the leaking of any gastric contents from the tube during its removal.
    Intervention - ______________________________

Nutritional Substances

Provide an example of a source for each of the following nutritional substances.

27. Trace element - ________________
28. Mineral - ____________________
29. Cholesterol - __________
30. Protein - __________
31. Complex carbohydrate - __________
32. Iodine - __________
33. High fiber food - __________
34. Monosaccharide - __________
35. Polyunsaturated - __________
36. Potassium - __________

Additional Enrichment Activities

1. Interview a person who is a member of a weight loss program such as Weight Watchers. Find out what they are eating, what is difficult for them, what is easy, and what is encouraging for them.
2. Plan a diet for a patient who is restricted in his cholesterol and saturated fat intake.
3. Do a 24-hour recall of your food and fluid intake and point out improvements for a balanced diet.

Suggested Readings

Blackburn GL, et al: Aspects of nutritional counseling. Hospital Medicine 23(1):100-1+, 1987.

Heins JM, et al: The new look in diabetic diets. American J Nursing 87(2):196-98, 1987

Holmes R, et al: Nutrition know-how: combating pressure sores-nutritionally. American J Nursing 87(10):1301-03, 1987

Stephenson MA: Meeting America's 1990 nutrition goals: we'll need a strong finish. FDA Consumer 21(7):15-7, 1987.

Computer Assisted Instruction

Sugar. Media Distributors

Food facts. MECC

Dietary interventions in the control of hypertension. Medi-Sim, Inc.

Nutritional assessment of the pregnant woman. Medi-Sim, Inc.

Chapter 32
Bowel Elimination

In Chapter 32 of Fundamentals of Nursing (Taylor, 1988) the physiology of bowel elimination and the many factors that influence the process of elimination are presented. Selected nursing diagnoses of common bowel elimination patterns are explored, and focused assessment, planning, implementation, and evaluation strategies are discussed. Because nurses frequently encounter clients with disorders that affect the bowel, students will find the information in this chapter essential to assisting clients cope with illnesses, diagnostic tests, or pharmacologic agents that affect bowel functioning.
After studying this chapter and completing the workbook exercises, the learner should be able to

- Define key terms used in the chapter.
- Describe the physiology of bowel elimination.
- Identify ten variables that influence bowel elimination.
- Assess bowel elimination using appropriate interview questions and physical assessment skills.
- Assist with the following diagnostic measures: stool collection for laboratory analysis and direct and indirect visualization studies of the gastrointestinal tract.
- Develop nursing diagnoses that correctly identify bowel elimination problems amenable to nursing therapy.
- Demonstrate how to (1) promote regular bowel habits (timing, positioning, privacy, nutrition, exercise); (2) use cathartics, laxatives, and antidiarrheals; (3) empty the colon of feces (enemas, rectal suppositories, rectal catheters, digital removal of stools); (4) design and implement bowel training programs; and (5) use comfort measures to ease defecation.
- Plan, implement, and evaluate nursing care related to select nursing diagnoses involving bowel problems.

Key Terms Chapter 32

The learner will want to become famaliar with the following key terms used in Chapter 32 prior to attempting the workbook exercises.

bowel movement
bowel training program
cathartic
chyme
colon
constipation
diarrhea
endoscopy
enema
feces
flatulence
flatus
hemorrhoids
impaction (fecal)
incontinence (fecal)
laxative
occult blood
ostomy
peristalsis
stoma
stool
suppository

Elimination: Match

Match each of the following terms with the appropriate definition.

Definitions:

A. sounds produced by hyperactive intestinal peristalsis
B. hidden quantity only detectable by chemical testing
C. sound caused by excess flatus trapped in the intestine
D. breakdown of the epidermis
E. direct visualization of the lining of a hollow organ using a scope
F. induces emptying of the GI tract
G. as in the intestine that is passed through the rectum
H. inability of anal sphincter to control discharge
I. an artificial opening of an internal organ of the surface of the body created by surgery
J. opening into the body created for excretion of body wastes

Terms:

1. _____ cathartic
2. _____ endoscopy
3. _____ flatulence
4. _____ incontinence
5. _____ occult blood
6. _____ ostomy
7. _____ borborygmus
8. _____ stoma
9. _____ excoriation
10. _____ hyperresonance

Large Intestine: Completion

Fill in the blanks of the paragraph below concerning the physiology of the large intestine.

The large intestine extends from the (11) ____________________ _______________ to the (12)______________________________. It varies in its width but it can be as wide as (13)______________inch(es) and as narrow as (14)______________inch(es). It absorbs as much as (15)____________ cc to (16)___________ cc of water from the waste products to form the normal stool. The (17)_________________ contains feces ready for excretion. These empty into the (18)______________ and through the (19)________ _______. The (20)________________ muscles control the discharge of feces and gas. The innervation of the (21)________________ nervous system makes the act of (22)____________________ under both involuntary and voluntary control.

Bowel Elimination : Case Study

Mr. John Cranby, age 70 years old, suffers from constipation intermittently, especially when under stress. He doesn't like fruit and drinks very little water. He is in the hospital for diagnostic studies of a spot on his lung and his nurses noted that he hadn't had a bowel movement in 5 days, was distended, and complained of extreme discomfort because of his lack of a bowel movement. Please write (1) your nursing diagnosis, (2) client goals and (3) nursing interventions based on his patient profile.

23. Nursing diagnosis

____

____

24. Client Goals

A. ____

____

B. ____

____

25. Nursing Interventions

____

____

____

____

____

____

Bowel Elimination : Crossword Puzzle

Across

15. Bran, whole wheat & apples are good sources of this
25. Test for occult blood in stool
54. Indole and skatole cause this in stool
58. Complication of bowel paralysis post operatively
64. Can cause percussed hyperresonance
97. Contraction of circular & longitudinal muscles of intestine
130. Ideal position for client during enema administration
138. This part of autonomics inhibits movement of intestines
153. Common laxative (abrv)
194. Constipation is side effect of this drug
223. Last part of large intestine
237. Treatment that soothes the perineal area

Down

9. Maneuver used in aiding defecation
16. Will change color of stools to black
21. Growth prone to cancer of colon
33. Study of esophagus and stomach (abrv)
56. Opening for the use of water elimination
98. May be needed for the constipated client
138. Excreted feces
148. Received by large intestine from small intestine
153. These impulses carried by sympathetics that innervate the internal sphincter
180. The outlet of the rectum
188. A lot of this helps prevent constipation

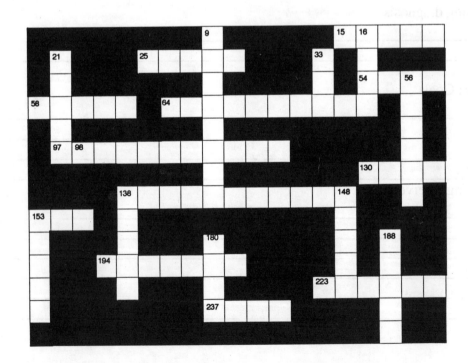

Bowel Elimination Problem Identification

Please identify a problem of bowel elimination with each of the following statements/quotes and/or descriptions.

26. Three days post-operatively - abdominal distention - no bowel sounds - vomiting even with presence of nasogastric tube

    ____

27. Pressure of liquid fecal seepage - extreme distention - no normal bowel movement for 6 days in an elderly patient

    ____

28. Encourage low fiber content in this client who has lost both fluid and electrolyte. If to an extreme degree may need intravenous fluid replacement

    ____

29. "I was so uncomfortable after eating that Mexican food last evening. I guess I ate too many beans and drank too much beer. How embarrassing!"

    ____

30. Mrs. John is so humiliated when this happens, but she can't seem to help herself and call the nurse in time before the bed is soiled

    ____

Enema Classification

Please identify the classification of each enema:
Cleansing, Retention or *Return Flow* (***C, R,*** or ***RF***).

31. Harris Flush - ______________
32. Carminative - ______________
33. Soap suds - ______________
34. Tap water - ______________
35. Oil retention - ______________
36. Hypertonic - ______________

GI Jeopardy

Please respond to the following statements with a sentence in the form of a question.

37. A special tube that can be used for clients with uncontrollable diarrhea.
What is a
____

38. These are abnormally distended veins commonly found in a client with constipation.
What are
____

39. Water can hinder the testing of this specimen.
What is
____

40. They come to the anal area during the night and retreat into the anal canal during the day.
What are
____

41. A flexible, fiberoptic scope will show the lining of the esophagus, stomach and duodenum.
What is an
____

42. Foods with skins, seeds and shells are to be avoided.
What are
____

43. The use of this laxative may decrease absorption of fat soluble vitamins and some drugs and cause lipid pneumonia if aspirated.
What is
____

44. The client is instructed to retain this for at least 30 minutes.
What is an
____

45. Introduce this well beyond the internal sphincter so it is in the rectum.
What is a
____

46. The color of this part of bowel anatomy should be dark pink to red.
What is a
____

47. This treatment is not done on ileostomies because fecal content is liquid and cannot be controlled.
What is an
____

Additional Enrichment Activities

1. Visit your local cancer association to acquire some brochures on clients with ostomies. Evaluate the brochures for knowledge/information and as a tool for patient teaching.
2. Spend a day in X-ray and observe all the GI diagnostic tests. Be alert for not only how the tests are performed, but to the patient's physiologic and psychosocial responses.

3. Spend a day in the GI lab to observe endoscopies. Again consider both the procedure and the patient's responses.
4. Make rounds with the ostomy nurse to become better informed about what she/he does and to observe the needs and reactions of patients with ostomies.
5. Do a role play with your fellow classmate with the scenario being you as a nurse and your partner as your client getting prepared for her colostomy surgery the next day.
6. Write out your feelings and problems you could foresee if you had to have an ileostomy done. Go through a week's activities post-surgery.
7. Make arrangements with your instructor for you to observe colon surgery.
8. Research the training needed for an ostomy clinician.

Suggested Readings for Bowel Elimination

Basch, A: Changes in elimination...associated with cancer. Seminars in Oncology Nursing 3(4):287-292, 1987

Brucker, MC: Management of common minor discomforts in pregnancy: managing gastrointestinal problems in pregnancy. J Nurse Midwifery 33(2):67-73, 1988

Clarke, B: Making sense of enemas. Nursing Times 84(30):40-41, 1988

Ellickson, EB: Bowel management for the homebound elderly. J Gerontogical Nursing 14(1):16-19, 1988

Groth, F: Effects of wheat bran in the diet of postsurgical orthopaedic patients to prevent constipation. Orthopaedic Nursing 7(4):41-46, 1988

Hagisawa, S et al: Effects of posture during defecation using a bedpan and a bedside commode on heart rate and oxygen consumption in normal adults. Progress in Cardiovascular Nursing 3(1):7-12, 1988

Hahn, K: Think twice about diarrhea. Nursing 17(9):78-80, 1987

McShane, RE et al: Constipation: impact of etiological factors. J Gerontological Nursing 14(4):31-34, 1988

Performing GI Procedures. Nursing Photobook. Horsham, PA, Intermed Communications, Inc. 1981

Saltzstein, RJ et al: Anorectal injuries incident to enema adminstration: a recurring avoidable problem. American J of Physical Medicine and Rehabilitation 67(4):186-188, 1988

Smith, CE: Investigating absent bowel sounds. Nursing 17(11):73, 76-77, 1987

Smith, LG: Home treatment of mild, acute diarrhea and secondary dehydration of infants and small children: an educational program for parents in a shelter for the homeless. J Professional Nursing 4(1):60-63, 1988

Sondheimer, JM: Resolving chronic constipation in children. Patient Care 21(5):108-112, 1987

Vargas, J: Sorting out the causes of vomiting and diarrhea. Emergency Medicine 20(3):138-142, 1988

Computer Assisted Instruction

Patients who need help with GI function. Simulated Patient Encounters in Medical-Surgical Nursing. J.B.Lippincott Company

Chapter 33
Urinary Elimination

Physiology of the urinary tract and the multiple factors affecting urinary elimination are explored in this chapter. The nursing process is presented with a focus on nursing diagnoses common to urinary problems (Taylor, 1988).

After studying this chapter and completing the workbook exercises, the learner should be able to

- Define the key terms used in the chapter.
- Describe the physiology of the urinary system.
- Identify seven variables that influence urination.
- Assess urinary elimination, using appropriate interview questions and physical assessment skills.
- Execute the following assessment measures: measure urine output, collect urine specimens, determine the presence of select abnormal urine constituents, determine urine specific gravity, and assist with diagnostic tests and procedures.
- Develop nursing diagnoses that correctly identify urinary problems amenable to nursing therapy.
- Demonstrate how to promote normal urination; facilitate use of the toilet, bedpan, urinal, and commode; perform catheterization; and assist with urinary diversions.
- Plan, implement, and evaluate nursing care related to select nursing diagnoses involving urinary problems.

Key Terms Used in Chapter 33

Prior to beginning the workbook exercises for Chapter 33 of the Fundamentals of Nursing textbook, the learner will want to become familiar with the following key terms.

anuria
catheter
condom catheter
cystoscopy
dysuria
enuresis
Foley catheters
frequency
functional incontinence
glycosuria
hematuria
hesitancy
hydrometer
ileal conduit
incontinence
indwelling urethral catheter
intravenous pyelogram
irrigation
micturition
nocturia
oliguria
orthostatic albuminuria
pneumaturia
polyuria
proteinuria
pyuria
reflex incontinence
residual urine
retention
retrograde pyelogram
stoma
stress incontinence
suprapubic catheter
suppression
total incontinence
micturition
nocturia
oliguria
orthostatic albuminuria
pneumaturia
polyuria
proteinuria
pyuria
reflex in continence
residual urine
retention
retrograde pyelogram
stoma
stress incontinence
suprapubic catheter
suppression
total incontinence
urination
urge incontinence
urgency
urinometer
voiding

Urinary System Diagnostic Procedures: Match

Match the following diagnostic procedures with their definition. You may use the same word more than once.

A. Cystoscopy
B. Intravenous Pyelogram
C. Retrograde Pyelogram

1. _____ Involves injection of IV contrast material
2. _____ Contrast material is injected into renal pelvis via ureter
3. _____ Dysuria and hematuria may occur following the procedure
4. _____ Instrument used to provide direct visualization of bladder
5. _____ A signed consent is required for the procedure
6. _____ May cause skin rash, nausea or hives
7. _____ Nosocomial infection can occur following procedure

Urinary Medication: Completion

Describe how the following types of medications affect urination.

8. Diuretics:

____

9. Cholinergics:

____

10. Analgesics:

____

11. Tranquilizers:

____

Urine Collection: Completion

The following statements refer to the collection of urine specimen. Please complete the blanks.

12. A _________ urine specimen is not required for a routine urinalysis.
13. Urine which is allowed to stand at room temperature for a long period of time may alter the _________ of urine.
14. Sterile urine specimens may be obtained using the _________ technique, by _______ the client, or by obtaining the specimen from an _________ already in place.
15. When collecting a 24-hour urine, it is important to collect _________ of the urine voided in a full ___________ period.
16. When collecting a mid-stream or clean-catch specimen, the client ___________ a little, the specimen is then collected ___________ and both the beginning and end voidings are ____________.
17. A mid-stream voided specimen from a male is ____________.
18. A freshly voided urine specimen is required when determining the presence of _______ or ______________.
19. The purpose for the client urinating and discarding the urine 30 minutes prior to the collection of a double voided specimen is to insure elimination of urine which has ____________ in the _____________ since the last voiding.
20. The nurse may collect urine samples and perform tests on the urine for the presence of _________, ___________, ___________, or _____________.
21. Urine specimens must be collected from the indwelling catheter rather than the ______ _________ to ensure a fresh specimen and accurate _________________.

Urinary Elimination Crossword Puzzle

IV. Complete the crossword puzzle below.

ACROSS:

1. Increased incidence of voiding
2. Excessive urinary output
3. Desire to void
4. Strong desire to void
5. Artificial opening for waste excretion
6. Tube used for urine drainage from bladder
7. No urine voided
8. Difficulty in voiding
9. Ureters connected to ileum with a stoma on the abdominal wall
10. Inability to retain urine after the age of toilet training

DOWN:

1. Involuntary urination during the night
2. Procedure to visualize the urinary bladder
3. Incontinence occurring when a specific bladder volume is reached
4. Frequency of urination at night
5. Delay or difficulty in initiating voiding
6. Flushing the bladder with solution
7. Stoppage of urine production
8. Pus in the urine

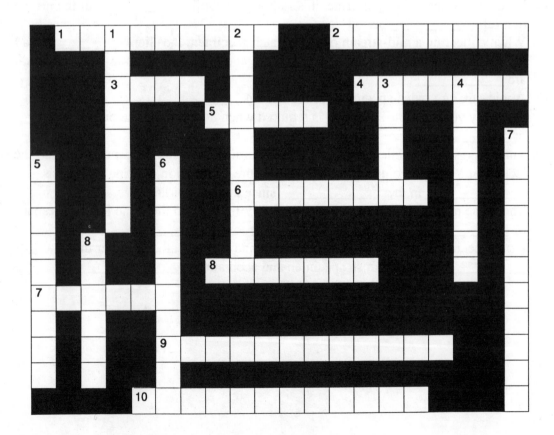

Urinary Terms: Word Scramble and Definition

The following are terms used for common urinary problems. Unscramble the terms, and define each one.

22. **syiguloacr:**____
23. **sohrtactoti muruilbanai:**______________________________
24. **reathuiem:**____
25. **netorietn:**____
26. **eionpiurtar:**____
27. **giorauli:**____
28. **tpmrnaueaii:**____
29. **ryduasi:**____

Incontinence: Match

Match the following types of incontinence with their definition or cause.

Definitions/Cause:

30. _____ Related to overdistention of bladder
31. _____ Involuntary, unpredictable urination
32. _____ Related to decreased bladder capacity
33. _____ Involuntary urination at somewhat predictable intervals
34. _____ Loss of urine occurring with increased abdominal pressure
35. _____ Continuous and unpredictable loss of urine
36. _____ Related to spinal cord, disease or trauma
37. _____ Involuntary urination following a strong urge to urinate
38. _____ Related to altered environment
39. _____ Related to bladder spasms.

Type of incontinence:

A. reflex incontinence
B. total incontinence
C. urge incontinence
D. stress incontinence
E. functional incontinence

Urinary Elimination Definition of Terms

Define the following terms:

40. Hydrometer:____
41. Micturition:____
42. Residual Urine:____________________________________
43. Suprapubic Catheter:_______________________________
44. Urinometer:____
45. Voiding:____
46. Foley Catheter:____________________________________

Characteristics of Urine

List the normal characteristics of urine

47. ____
48. ____
49. ____
50. ____
51. ____
52. ____

Additional Enrichment Activities:

1. In the clinical agency, observe the nurse collect various urine samples and label them for the laboratory. If possible include:
    a. specimen from a foley catheter
    b. a sterile specimen
    c. a double voided specimen
    d. a clean catch specimen
2. If possible, visit the laboratory at your clinical agency and observe the various tests that are performed on urine specimens.
3. Teach a client how to collect a clean-catch urine specimen.

Suggested Readings

Andersen M. et al: Collecting a reliable urine specimen for drug analysis. J Nursing Administration 17(1):25,32, 1987

Conti MT, et al: Preventing UTIs--what works? American J Nursing87(3):307-9, 1987

Cefalu CA: Management of the bedridden patient with irreversible urinary incontinence. 23(6):83-7, 1987.

Micturition: Innervation and physiologic considerations. 23(2):144+, 1987

Computer Assisted Instruction

Gomez SP: Patients who need help with urinary elimination. Simulated Patient Encounters in Medical-Surgical Nursing. J.B.Lippincott Company

Chapter 34
Oxygenation

Chapter 34 of Fundamentals of Nursing (Taylor, 1988) presents the physiology of oxygenation, identifies factors which influence respiratory function, and describes aspects of nursing process pertinent to care of clients with respiratory problems.
After studying Chapter 34 and completing the workbook exercises, the student should be able to

- Define key terms used in the chapter.
- Describe the principles of respiratory physiology.
- Describe age-related differences that influence care of the client with respiratory problems.
- Identify six factors that influence respiratory function.
- Perform a comprehensive respiratory assessment using appropriate interview questions and physical assessment skills.
- Develop nursing diagnoses that correctly identify problems that may be treated by independent nursing interventions.
- Describe 11 nursing strategies to promote adequate respiratory functioning, identifying their rationale.
- Plan, implement, and evaluate nursing care related to select nursing diagnoses involving respiratory problems.

Key Terms Chapter 34

You will want to become familiar with the meaning of the following key terms used in this chapter prior to beginning the workbook exercises.

atelectasis
bronchodilator
bronchoscope
bronchoscopy
congestion
cupping
cystologic study
fremitus
endoscopy
expectorant
expiratory reserve volume
forced vital capacity
functional residual capacity
hemoptysis
hyperventilation
hypoventilation
hypoxia
inspiratory reserve volume
laryngoscope
laryngoscopy
lozenge
nonproductive cough
percussion
perfusion
phlegm
postural drainage
productive cough
radiography
rales
residual volume
rhonchi
skin test
spirometer
suppressant
sympathomimetic agent
tidal volume
total lung capacity
thoracentesis
ventilation
vibration
vital capacity

Key Terms: Match

Please match the following key terms with their appropriate definitions.

Terms:

1. ___ atelectasis
2. ___ hemoptysis
3. ___ percussion
4. ___ rales
5. ___ spirometer
6. ___ bradypnea
7. ___ hyperventilation
8. ___ thoracentesis
9. ___ cupping
10. ___ lozenge

Definitions:

A. Non-continuous sounds produced by delayed reopening of deflated airways
B. Increased rate and depth of ventilation above normal
C. Collapse of lung tissue preventing gaseous exchange
D. Manual percussion of lung areas to loosen pulmonary secretions
E. Aspiration of fluid from the plural space
F. Small solid medication that is held in mouth and relieves cough through a local anesthetic action
G. Coughing up bloody sputum
H. Resonance is heard over the normal lung when this is performed
I. Abnormally slow rate of breathing
J. Instrument that measures and records volume of inspired and expired air

The Nursing Examination of the Respiratory System

Please complete the following by filling in the blanks.

Inspection

11. On inspection of the chest the __________ - __________ diameter should be less than the __________ diameter and during respirations, the movement of the chest should be __________________.

Palpation

12. The _________________ should be equidistant from each clavicle and when measuring respiratory excursion with both hands on client's posterior thorax, the thumbs should move __________________ to __________________ cm on maximal inspiration.

Percussion

13. During percussion of the normal lung, __________________ is heard. On the other hand, in the client with emphysema, ______________ is heard. When fluid replaces lung tissue, the area over it elicits _________________________ when percussed.

Auscultation

14. The client should breathe ____________ ___________ ____________ ___________ when the nurse is auscultating because ______________ breathing produces false abnormal breath sounds. Another term for abnormal breath sounds is ____________ sound.

Oxygen Treatment

Name the oxygen treatment described by the following brief statements.

15. Most commonly used oxygen delivery aid. ______________________
16. Gastric distention can occur with this because oxygen flow can inadvertently enter the stomach. __________________
17. The client will rebreathe about one third of the expired air from the reservoir bag with this device. __________________
18. This device can provide the highest concentration of oxygen to the client who is breathing spontaneously. __________________
19. A physician will often use this for a client with COPD to provide him with an exact concentration of oxygen. ____________________________
20. Today, it's only used for pediatric clients who need cool and highly humidified air flow because it doesn't maintain precise O2 concentration. ___________________

Pulmonary Function Tests

Please write a brief description of each of the following pulmonary function tests and include the normal values.

21. Tidal Volume -______________________________
22. Inspiratory Reserve Volume (IRV) - ____________________
23. Expiratory Reserve Volume (ERV) - ____________________
24. Vital Capacity (VC) - ____________________________
25. Forced Vital Capacity (FVC) - ________________________
26. Functional Residual Capacity (FRC) - ____________________
27. Residual Volume (RV) - ____________________________
28. Total Lung Capacity (TLC) - __________________________

Respiratory Crossword Puzzle

Across

20. Circulation of blood
81. Adventitious lung sound
93. Breathing treatment (abrv)
115. Air inspired beyond the normal breath
150. Process of treating or combining with oxygen (abrv)
179. Diagnostic test to see lung fields
201. Difficulty breathing
225. Organism often cultured in pneumonia
234. Abnormal sounds heard on inspiration

Down

6. Exam of bronchi through a scope
11. Exchange of O2 & CO2 between this and blood
25. Hazardous to your health
35. Decreased amount of oxygen
77. Treatment to loosen lung secretions
81. Air in the lungs after maximum expiration (abrv)
181. Steroid used frequently for lung inflammation
203. Type of charting
207. Measurement of pH, pCO2 and pO2

6 11 20 25 35 77 81 93 115 150 179 181 201 203 207 225 234

Respiratory Jeopardy

Please answer the following statements in the form of a question.

29. It lies between the parietal and visceral pleurae.
    Question: ______________________________
30. Gases move passively from an area of higher concentration to one of lower concentration.
    Question : ______________________________
31. This is a movement of air in and out of the lungs.
    Question: ______________________________
34. Millions of these make up the lungs.
    Question: ______________________________
35. This is an important tool in the early steps of the nursing process of the respiratory client.
    Question: ______________________________
36. This auscultated sound is caused by inflammation of pleural surfaces.
    Question: ______________________________
37. Ineffective airway clearance.
    Question: ______________________________
38. These drugs will facilitate removal of respiratory secretions by reducing secretion viscosity.
    Question: ______________________________
39. This tube goes through the nose or mouth into the trachea.
    Question: ______________________________
40. A is for airway, B is for breathing, C is for circulation.
    Question : ______________________________
41. The correct ratio of compressions to ventilations is 5:1.
    Question: ______________________________
42. Antigens are injected into the skin to note an antibody response.
    Question: ______________________________

Additional Enrichment Activities

1. Make a visit to your local lung association and become familiar with the free AV materials on hand which could be used for patient/family education. Make a list of the materials to share with classmates.
2. Make arrangements to spend a day with a respiratory nurse clinician in a local hospital. Become acquainted with his/her nursing role and the kind of clients with whom s/he works.
3. Attend a class for people trying to stop smoking at one of the local hospitals' stop smoking clinics. Talk with them about their smoking habit and the difficulties/joys they are experiencing as they work on stopping.

4. Arrange with your nursing instructor to observe a client having lung surgery.
5. Accompany a respiratory therapist as he/she makes rounds. Note the various kinds of clients (i.e., diagnoses) and interventions/treatments given.
6. Observe a client having pulmonary function studies. Note not only the procedure(s) but the needs and reactions of the clients.
7. Assist a respiratory therapist or nurse in drawing an arterial blood gas sample. Compare the results obtained with what you know/observe about the patient.
8. Spend some time in a respiratory ICU and observe the clients on ventilators. What are some of their special needs (physiological, psychosocial, spiritual)?
9. Arrange with your instructor to observe a bronchoscopy. Note not only the procedure but the needs/reactions of the patient. Explore how having observed this procedure will make a difference in how you will prepare a patient for this procedure in the future.
10. Spend some time in X-ray observing respiratory diagnostic tests such as chest x-ray, lung scan, tomogram, etc.

Suggested Readings

Ahrens TS, Rutherford KA: The new pulmonary math applying the a/a ratio. American J Nursing 87(3):337-40, 1987

Kim MJ, et al: Ineffective airway clearance and ineffective breathing patterns: theoretical and research base for nursing diagnosis. Nursing Clinics of North America 22(1):125-34, 1987

Stevens MS: Fine tuning your chest PT. American J Nursing 87(12):1566-72, 1987

Computer Assisted Instruction

Nursing Electronic Workbook: Respiratory Assessment (9 programs reviewing respiratory assessment) Vockell Software.

Chapter 35
Fluid, Electrolyte, and Acid-Base Balance

Chapter 35 of Fundamentals of Nursing (Taylor, 1988) provides opportunity for the learner to acquire basic knowledge of fluid, electrolyte, and acid-base balance. Focused learning experiences are provided in which the nursing process is demonstrated in clinical context with surgical and oncology clients.

After studying this chapter and completing the workbook exercises the learner should be able to

- Define key terms used in the chapter.
- Describe the functions of body fluids, the two main compartments where fluids are located in the body, and factors that affect variations in fluid compartments.
- Describe the functions, sources and losses, and regulation of main electrolytes of the body.
- Explain the principles of osmosis, diffusion, active transport, and filtration.
- Describe how thirst and the organs of homeostasis function to maintain fluid homeostasis.
- Describe the role of buffer systems, and specific respiratory and renal mechanisms in achieving acid-base balance.
- Identify the etiologies, defining characteristics, and treatment modalities for common fluid, electrolyte, and acid-base disturbances.
- Perform a comprehensive fluid, electrolyte, and acid-base balance assessment.
- Describe the role of dietary modification, modification of fluid intake, medication administration, intravenous therapy, blood replacement, and total parenteral nutrition in resolving fluid, electrolyte, and acid-base imbalances.
- Plan, implement, and evaluate nursing care related to select nursing diagnoses involving fluid, electrolyte and acid-base imbalances.

Key Terms Chapter 35

The learner will want to become familiar with the key terms used in this chapter prior to attempting the workbook exercises.

acid
acidosis
active transport
agglutinin
alkali
alkalosis
anion
antibody
antigen
base
blood transfusion
buffer
cation
cellular fluid
colloid osmotic pressure
crossmatching
dehydration
diffusion
donor
edema
electrolyte
embolus
extracellular fluid
filtration
filtration pressure
fluid volume deficit
fluid volume excess
hydration
hydrostatic pressure
hypercalcemia
hyperkalemia
hypermagnesemia
hypernatremia
hyperphosphatemia
hypervolemia
hypocalcemia
hypokalemia
hypomagnesemia
hyponatremia
hypophosphatemia
insensible water loss
interstitial fluid
intracellular fluid
intravascular fluid
intravenous fluid
ion
ionization
metabolic acidosis
metabolic alkalosis
milliequivalent
milliliter
nonelectrolyte
oncotic pressure
osmolality
osmoreceptors
osmosis
osteomalacia
pH
phlebitis
respiratory acidosis
respiratory alkalosis
Rh
solute
solvent
speed shock
third-space fluid shift
total body water
total parenteral nutrition
typing

Functions of Water

List 5 of the primary functions of water in the body.

1. ______________________________
2. ______________________________
3. ______________________________
4. ______________________________
5. ______________________________

Function and Regulation Properties of Electrolytes

Place the correct electrolyte symbol in the blanks.

Functions:

6.___ Maintains isotonicity of body fluids

7.___ Needed for Vitamin B absorption

8.___ Essential for hydrochloric acid production in gastric juices

9.___ With carbonic acid, forms body's primary buffer system

10.___ Vital role in transmission of electrical impulses, especially in nerve, heart and skeletal muscle tissue

Regulation by:

11.___ Calcitonin and parathyroid hormone (PTH)

12.___ Paired with Na+ and excreted by the kidneys

13.___ Aldosterone stimulates the kidneys to conserve through reabsorption

14.___ Parathyroid hormone and activated Vitamin D

Organs of Homeostasis: Matching

Match the organ of homeostasis with its function by inserting the correct letter in the appropriate blank.

Organ:

15. _____ lungs
16. _____ pituitary gland
17. _____ parathyroid glands
18. _____ kidneys
19. _____ heart and blood vessels
20. _____ adrenal glands

Function:

a. Regulate oxygen and carbon dioxide levels of the blood.
b. Regulates calcium and phosphate.
c. Contain stretch receptors which react to hypovolemia by stimulating fluid retention.
d. Selectively retain electrolytes and water; excrete metabolic wastes, primarily acids.
e. Regulate K+ and Na+ by secretion of aldosterone.
f. Stores and releases antidiuretic hormone, which causes water retention.

Acid-Base Sentence: Completion

Complete these sentences about acid-base balance by supplying the missing word in the blank provided.

21. The kidneys form ________ salts by exchanging a Na+ ion for a H+ ion when ______________ sodium phosphate is converted to ______________ sodium phosphate.
22. In the lungs, carbon dioxide and water are acted upon by carbonic anhydrase to produce ______________________.
23. The kidneys regulate the concentration of bicarbonate in the plasma through the production of__________________ in the kidney tubules. It unites with hydrogen and chloride for excretion as __________________.
24. In addition to the regulatory mechanism in Item 25, the kidneys control H+ balance by forming additional ________________________ as needed, and by excreting __________________ ions.
25. Respiratory acidosis and alkalosis are caused by __________________ disturbances/phenomena. This alters the ____________________ proportion. Primary compensatory organs are the ____________________.
26. Metabolic acidosis and alkalosis are caused by ____________ disturbances/phenomena. This alters the ______________________ proportion. Primary compensatory organs are the ______________________.

Acid-Base Balance Compensatory Terms

Supply the correct diagnostic label and/or compensatory term for each acid-base balance described in the left column. The compensatory terms are provided in the right column. Some compensatory terms may be used more than once.

Acid-base balance:

27. In ______________________, the extracellular fluid contains proportionately too much bicarbonate. To compensate, respirations become slow and shallow in an attempt to retain ________________, and the kidneys attempt to excrete _____, _____, and _____, and retain _____ and _____.

28. In _______________, there is a proportionate deficit of carbonic acid in the extra-cellular fluid, due to increased alveolar ventilation. Compensation is achieved by ________; the kidneys also excrete more _______ and retain more _______.

Diagnostic label/Compensatory Terms:

Respiratory Acidosis
Respiratory Alkalosis
Metabolic Acidosis
Metabolic Alkalosis
H+
Carbon Dioxide
Bicarbonate
Ammonium
K+
Na+
Carbonic acid
Hypoventilation

29. _____________ is a proportionate excess of carbonic acid in the extracellular fluid, usually caused by a ventilation problem. To compensate, the rate and depth of respirations increases, in an effort to "blow off" _____________. The kidneys attempt to retain _____ and increase their excretion of _____.

30. _____________ is a proportionate deficit of bicarbonate in the extracellular fluid. The lungs attempt to compensate by excreting ___________, so the rate and depth of respirations increases. The kidneys attempt to retain _________ and excrete more _________________________.

Nursing Implications of IV Therapy: Matching

The nurse is responsible for measures to prevent complications of IV therapy, and for instituting the proper action should a complication occur. Match the correct preventive or treatment measures to the complications below. Some items may be used more than once.

Complications:

A. Speed shock
B. Phlebitis
C. Embolus
D. Fluid overload
E. Thrombus
F. Infiltration
G. Infection

Preventive Measures:

31. ____ Limit the movement of the extremity with the IV.
32. ____ Use microdrip on pediatric clients.
33. ____ Monitor the flow rate carefully & often.
34. ____ Do not allow air to enter the infusion line.
35. ____ Use aseptic technique when starting infusion

If symptoms occur, the nurse should initiate treatment measures:

36. ____ Discontinue the infusion if symptoms occur.
37. ____ Apply warm, moist compresses to the affected site.
38. ____ Report to M.D. any sudden pain or breathing difficulty.
39. ____ If symptoms develop, slow rate of infusion
40. ____ Restart the infusion at another site.

Additional Enrichment Activities

1. Go to the clinical unit and find at least 3 client charts in which abnormal electrolyte lab values are reported. For each client, attempt to find reported/charted clinical signs and symptoms that would correlate with the abnormal electrolyte value(s). Identify the specific nursing diagnoses and plan of care that has been established based upon the electrolyte abberation.

2. Visit a community blood bank. Find out what is done (a) to insure that an adequate community blood supply is available, (b) to protect the blood supply from contamination, and (c) to addresss concerns related to AIDS. Write a paragraph (a) explaining how much a unit of blood costs, how long it can be kept; (b) explaining what autologous blood transfusion is; how it is accomplished, and how much it costs.

Suggested Readings

Chenevy B: Overview of fluid and electrolytes. Nursing Clinics of North America 22(4):749-760, 1987

Poyss, AS: Assessment and nursing diagnosis of fluid and electrolyte disorders. Nursing Clinics of North America 22(4)773-784, 1987

Schwartz MW: Potassium Imbalances, American J of Nursing 87(10):1292-1299, 1987

Unit VIII
Promoting Healthy Psychosocial Responses

Holistic client care, focusing on self-concept, sensory stimulation, sexuality, and spirituality, are the concepts discussed in the four chapters comprising Unit VIII. The intent of this unit is to provide the learner with the knowledge base necessary for promoting healthy psychosocial responses in clients. Learners are encouraged to plan and implement nursing interventions which meet the needs and support the strengths of clients in health and illness.

Chapter 36
Self-Concept

Chapter 36 of Fundamentals of Nursing (Taylor, 1988) provides opportunity for the learner to acquire knowledge of the (1) dimensions of self-concept, (2) defense mechanisms, and (3) key factors affecting self-concept.

After studying the chapter and completing the workbook exercises the learner should be able to

- Define key terms used in the chapter.
- Identify three dimensions of self-concept: self-knowledge, self-expectation, self-evaluation (self-esteem).
- Describe three major steps in the development of self-concept.
- Differentiate positive and negative self-concept and high and low self-esteem.
- Identify six variables that influence self-concept.
- Use appropriate interview questions and observations to asses a client's self-concept: self-knowledge (body image, client strengths), expectations, self-esteem (significance, role competence, virtue, power).
- Develop nursing diagnoses that correctly identify disturbances in self-concept (body image, self-esteem, role performance, self-identity).
- Describe nursing strategies that are effective in resolving self-concept problems.
- Plan, implement, and evaluate nursing care related to select nursing diagnoses for disturbances in self-concept.

Key Terms Chapter 36

Prior to attempting the workbook exercises for Chapter 36, the learner is advised to become familiar with the following key terms used in the chapter.

body image
competence
defense mechanisms
ideal self
power
self-actualization
self-concept
self-esteem
significance
social self
virtue

Assessment Data/Key Terms: Match

Place the letters corresponding to the key terms with the appropriate assessment data sentence .

Key Terms

BI Body Image
C Competence
DM Defense Mechanism
IS Ideal Self
P Power
S Significance
SA Self-Actualization
SS Social Self
V Virtue

Assessment Data

1. ____ An 18 year old girl who had an abortion said to the nurse, "I was wrong to have that abortion. I'm Catholic and God wouldn't want me to do that."
2. ____ An 83 year old resident in a nursing home raised 8 children on a farm in the Midwest. She stated to the nurse, "We did a good job of raising our children and I helped raise my sister's kids. Our family is real close and all the kids take good care of us. There's nothing like love in a family."
3. ____ The client in #2 above stated, "You know everyone loved Mr. and me 'cause we always helped our neighbors and everyone thought we had such good kids."
4. ____ Client in #2 and #3 above continued, "You know, honey, I think I was real good at sewing and gardening and making a home and teaching my children. That's really what God called me to do and it's important to find your niche and do it the best you can."
5. ____ Client in #2, #3, & #4 continued, "Now I couldn't be a nurse. I don't like hospitals, but I was sure a good wife and mother. I took care of our old parents and helped all our neighbors when they needed anything."
6. ____ A college student having difficulty with writing papers was instructed to correct and rewrite a term paper. The student's response was, "That teacher just wants to fail me because I let her know her tests aren't any good."

7. ____ A 19 year old male with chronic kidney failure screamed at the nurse, who asked for a urine specimen, "You all always want something and you think you really have it together. I could cause you real trouble if I wanted to."
8. ____A mother of three young children and the victim of physical abuse cried, "I wish I were like his sister. I'm a no good wife and mother and I never could cook or keep house."
9. ____An 11 year old girl, height 54 inches and weight 140 pounds, refused to play softball in gym class after other students called her "Roly-Poly" when she ran around the bases.

Self-Concept Order of Achievement

Rank from 1 to 6 in the order, from birth to death, in which achievement of a positive self-concept occurs.

10. ____ Incorporates into him/herself the parent's attitudes toward self.
11. ____ Internalizes the standards of society into self.
12. ____ Identifies with and tries out roles and behaviors of "heroes."
13. ____ Differentiates physical self from environment and others.
14. ____ Internalizes the attitudes of teachers and peers toward self.
15. ____ Has no self-concept.

Additional Enrichment Activities

1. Observe children ages 2-5 in a local nursery or preschool or church school for indications of self-concept development. Make a list of your observations to share with your class.
2. In the visit to observe 2-5 year olds (above), include observations of the environment and the children's interactions with peers and teachers. Note how these factors affect self-concept development.
3. Repeat Activities #1 and #2 for teenagers at a fast food restaurant or a high school or junior high lunch room.
4. Interview a person, 16-22 years old, whom you do not know. Explain that you are studying the development of self-concept in school and nothing they say will be repeated. You need not know their name. Ask the person to make a list of words describing them, their body, strengths, and weaknesses. (You will be assessing their self-knowledge.)
5. Follow-up on Activity #4 by asking the person you interview how he/she would like to be, would like to change or thinks he/she should be (self-ideal). Then assess the interviewee's overall self-esteem by comparing response to #4 and #5.

Suggested Readings

Schawib D et al: Nursing care of patients with an altered body image due to multiple sclerosis. Nursing Forum 22(2):72-76, 1985

Williamson MD: The nursing diagnosis of body image disturbance in adolescents dissatisfied with their physical characteristics. Holistic Nursing Practice 1(4):52-9, 1987

Chapter 37
Sensory Stimulation

Chapter 37 of Fundamentals of Nursing (Taylor, 1988) provides the learner with knowledge of (1) the process of sensation, (2) the role of the arousal mechanism, (3) sensory alterations, and (4) factors affecting sensory stimulation.

After studying this chapter and completing the workbook exercises, the learner should be able to

- Define key terms in the chapter.
- Describe the four conditions that must be met in each sensory experience.
- Explain the role of the reticular activating system in sensory experience.
- Identify etiologies and perceptual, cognitive, and emotional responses to sensory deprivation and sensory overload.
- Perform a comprehensive assessment of sensory functioning utilizing appropriate interview questions and physical assessment skills.
- Develop nursing diagnoses that correctly identify sensory-perceptual alterations that may be treated by independent nursing intervention.
- Describe specific nursing strategies to prevent sensory alterations, to stimulate the senses, and to assist clients with sensory difficulties.
- Develop a plan of nursing care to assist clients meet individualized sensory-perceptual goals.
- Implement individualized nursing strategies that successfully resolve the client's individualized sensory-perceptual alterations.
- Evaluate the plan of nursing care using specified criteria.

Key Terms Chapter 37

Prior to attempting the workbook exercises the student would be well advised to become familiar with the following key terms used in chapter 37.

arousal
auditory
gustatory
kinesthesia
olfactory
perception
reception
reticular activating system
sensoristasis
sensory deprivation
sensory overload
sensory-perceptual alterations
stimulus
tactile
visceral
visual

Sensory Status : Matching

Adequate assessment of sensory ability is often neglected by nursing staff. Draw a line from the sense being assessed, column one, to two methods of assessment on the right. Perform an actual assessment using each method.

***Method of Assessment*:**

1. ____Stand behind client and speak client's name in normal tone.
2. ____Ask client to identify a few grains of salt, then sugar, placed on the tongue.
3. ____Ask client to identify vinegar and alcohol held under nose.
4. ____Ask client to read aloud a newspaper or mail. Watch eye movement.
5. ____Alternating one or two dull points held 1/8" then 1/4", 1/2" or 1" apart (when client is blindfolded), ask client how many points touch skin.
6. ____Ask client to write name on a line or sew.
7. ____Stand behind client and ask in whisper, "Can you hear me?"
8. ____Ask client to identify perfume.
9. ____Ask client to identify few drops of lemon juice, then cocoa, placed on the tongue.
10 ____Ask client to put hand in bag or sack and remove on request a peanut, a safety pin and a rock.

Senses:

A. Vision
B. Hearing
C. Taste
D. Smell
E. Tactile

Impaired Senses : Matching

Persons with impaired sensation have high potential for injury. Match the letter indicating the impaired sense (Smell & Taste are together) with the following situations which are potentially dangerous or more dangerous because of the specific sensory deficit.

Increased Injury Potential:

11. ____ There is a fire alarm in the building which was sounded but Mable did not respond.
12. ____ George went to sleep while smoking in bed. He did not awaken although the mattress smoldered for hours before it burst into flame.
13. ____ Susan lived alone and kept everything in its place so she could find it. Friends visited,moved the furniture to talk, and Susan fell over a footstool after they left.
14. ____ Robert ate some left-over egg salad which looked good, but it made him very ill.
15. ____ Mary placed an electric heating pad, set on medium, on her 93 year old grandmother's feet. It burned the grandmother before she awoke.
16. ____ Steve had cataracts on both eyes. He had surgery on one eye, but he must wait for glasses. He stepped off of a curb and broke a hip.

Impaired Sense:

V Vision
H Hearing
S-T Smell-Taste
T Tactile

Additional Enrichment Activities

1. Select a resident in a local nursing home who has minimal hearing deficit and is described by the staff as "frequently confused". Interact with the person for 30 minutes on 5 consecutive days using as many sensory modalities as appropriate and possible. Compare the client's responses (cognitive, perceptual and emotional, see text page 1539) from your first and last visits and report any changes.
2. Eat one entire meal using salt-free and sugar-free foods with no added seasoning during preparation. Place cotton plugs in your nose while eating. Then, evaluate your perceptions of the meals.
3. Arrange for a "blind banquet" for your class. Have half the class go through the cafeteria line and eat while blindfolded. Have the other half of the class assist those who are blindfolded. Discuss reactions to this experience.
4. Place ear plugs in and ear muffs over your ears for 3 hours as you continue normal activity with others in your room or home. Describe your reactions to this experience.

Suggested Readings

Carver JA: Cataract Care Made Plain. American J of Nursing 87(5):626-30, 1987

Ophthalmic issues. Facts and Myths. AAOHN J 36(4):174-7, 1988

Parker P: Herman Snellen, 1834-1908. J Opthalmic Nurse Technology 7(1):38, 1988

Magilvy JK: Quality of Life of Hearing-Impaired Older Women. Nursing Research 34(3):140-44, 1985

Riley MAK: Nursing Care of the Client with Ear, Nose, and Throat Disorders. 356, New York, Springer Publishing Co., 1987

The loss of smell. Emergency Medicine, March 15, 20(5):104-6, 111-2, 114+, 1988

Chapter 38
Sexuality

Reproductive anatomy and physiology, the sexual response cycle, and factors that affect sexuality are the issues discussed in Chapter 38 of Fundamentals of Nursing (Taylor, 1988). The learner is provided with information about how to obtain a sexual history and appropriate interventions for nursing diagnoses that pertain to concerns with sexuality. After studying this chapter and completing the workbook exercises, the learner should be able to

- Define key terms used in the chapter.
- Describe male and female reproductive anatomy and physiology.
- Describe the sexual response cycle and differentiate between male and female responses.
- Identify and describe factors that affect an individual's sexuality.
- Perform a sexual assessment utilizing suggested interview questions and appropriate physical assessment skills.
- Describe types of sexual dysfunctions and assessment priorities for each one.
- Develop nursing diagnoses identifying a problem with sexuality that may be remedied by independent nursing actions.
- Describe five areas in which the nurse can provide the client with education to promote knowledge of sexuality.
- Plan, implement, and evaluate nursing care related to select nursing diagnoses involving problems of sexuality.

Key terms Chapter 38

Prior to beginning the workbook exercises the learner will want to become famaliar with the following terms used in the chapter.

abstinence
bisexuality
coitus
coitus interruptus
contraception
cunnilingus
dyspareunia
ejaculation
erectile failure
erection
erogenous zones
fellatio
fetishism
foreplay
gay
heterosexuality
homosexuality
impotence
Kegel exercises
lesbian
masochism
mastectomy
masturbation
menarche
menopause
menses
nocturnal emission
orgasm
orgasmic dysfunction
ovulation
ovum
pregnancy
premature ejaculation
rape
retarded ejaculation
sadism
sadomasochism
semen
sexual dysfunction
sexual intercourse
sexuality

Search-a-Word

The words that match the following definitions can be found going up, down, across, backwards and diagonally in the puzzle below.

1. ____________________ Auto Immune Deficiency Syndrome
2. ____________________ Breast Self Exam
3. ____________________ structure that connects the uterus and the vagina
4. ____________________ insertion of penis into the vagina
5. ____________________ stimulation of the female genitals by licking and sucking the clitoris and surrounding structures
6. ____________________ painful intercourse
7. ____________________ the expulsion of semen by the rhythmic contractions of the penis
9. ____________________ blood vessels in the shaft of the penis become congested
10. ____________________ stimulation of the male genitals by licking and sucking the penis and surrounding tissues
11. ____________________ sexual arousal with the aid of an inanimate object not generally associated with sexual activity
12. ____________________ a period of activity which stimulates coitus
13. ____________________ male homosexual

14. ____________________ erectile failure
15. ____________________ the promotion of good vaginal tone by localizing and strengthening the pubococcygeal muscles
16. ____________________ female homosexual
17. ____________________ the first menstrual period
18. ____________________ gaining sexual pleasure from the humiliation of being abused
19. ____________________ the cessation of a woman's menstrual activity, occurs between the ages of 45 to 55 yrs.
20. ____________________ menstrual flow
21. ____________________ the third phase of the sexual response
22. ____________________ day 14 when the mature ovum ruptures from the follicle and surface of the ovary and is swept into the fallopian tube
23. ____________________ Pelvic Inflammatory Disease
24. ____________________ the practice of gaining sexual pleasure while inflicting abuse on another person
25. ____________________ when sadism and masochism are practiced together
26. ____________________ a liquid consisting of seminal plasma and sperm
27. ____________________ the act of introducing the penis into the rectum
28. ____________________ the degree to which a person exhibits and experiences maleness or femaleness physically, emotionally, and mentally
29. ____________________ male fertilizing secretion
30. ____________________ Sexually Transmitted Disease
31. ____________________ organ that produces sperm and the hormones necessary for the maintenance of male characteristics
32. ____________________ pear-shaped female organ located between the urinary bladder and the rectum
33. ____________________ tubular, hollow organ that lies between the urinary urethra and the rectum in a female

```
A N O I T C E R E X I V R E C B B D
C D D E M F F G H Z Y X W V U U S T
T Y S R S E R Q P O N M M E N S E S
L S E D L L K J I H G S F E N E D E
E P I C A L P I D B I C D E I M F X
S A D O M A S O C H I S M G L E H U
B R Z I Y T X W S C D A K J I N N A
I E Q T P I O I C B S D A V N A O L
A U O U S O T P K O J I Y A G R I I
N N I S R E H G C V A S B G U C T T
F I E G F D T H C U B M A I S H A Y
Q A A R L S I S T L Z W C N O E L N
J S I A R S Q O E A P E F A D B U C
M W G Y M T F O U T E R U S O W C X
P E C N E T O P M I O T T O M M A E
K E I Y A L P E R O F S E N Y T J A
A H G S T P E M E N O P A U S E E N
```

Human Sexuality : Short Answer

Answer the following questions in the space provided.

34. How would you set the tone for taking a sexual history?

35. What is the best approach in obtaining useful information regarding your client's sexuality?

36. What are three questions you could use in obtaining a brief sexual history?

37. How would you address confidentiality?

38. Discuss some nursing interventions for assisting your client to develop an increased sexual desire.

39. Your 21 year old unmarried client is sexually active and is not using any contraceptives. Using the nursing process, how would you proceed?

40. Name elements of a sexual history for male and female clients.

41. Explain the PLISSIT

Additional Enrichment Activities

1. Practice self breast examor self testicular exam to become familiar with your normal tissue. Identify those who are at risk for breast cancer and testicular cancer.
2. Identify a nursing diagnosis having to do with your own sexuality (i.e. anxiety related to lack of information regarding sexually transmitted disease, or disturbance in body image related to body weight gain). Write both a short and long term goal along with a plan for resolution.
3. List ways in which you are a good role model in promoting healthy sexuality. Are there ways you could improve?

Suggested Readings

Brink PJ: Aspects of sexuality. Holistic Nursing Practice 1(4):12-20, 1987

Campsey JR: The sexual dimension of patient care. Nursing Forum 22(2):69-71, 1985

Woods NF: Toward a holistic perspective of human sexuality: alterations in sexual health and nursing diagnoses. Holistic Nursing Practice 1(4):1-11, 1987

Chapter 39
Spirituality

Spirituality is a significant dimension of a person's holistic being. This chapter of Fundamentals of Nursing (Taylor, 1988) provides the learner with a knowledge base of spirituality. In addition to suggestions for doing spiritual assessment, sample nursing diagnoses are developed for common problems of spiritual distress (spiritual pain, alienation, anxiety, guilt, anger, loss, and despair).

After studying this chapter and completing the workbook exercises, the learner should be able to

- Define key terms used in the chapter.
- Identify three spiritual needs believed to be common to all persons.
- Describe the influences of spirituality on everyday living, health, and illness.
- Differentiate life-affirming influences of religious beliefs from life-denying influences.
- Distinguish the spiritual beliefs and practices of the major religions practiced in the United States and Canada: Protestantism, Catholicism, Judaism.
- Identify five factors that influence spirituality.
- Perform a nursing assessment of spiritual health, utilizing appropriate interview questions and observation skills.
- Develop nursing diagnoses that correctly identify spiritual problems.
- Describe seven nursing stages to promote spiritual health and state their rationale.
- Plan, implement, and evaluate nursing care related to select nursing diagnoses involving spiritual problems.

Key Terms Chapter 39

Prior to beginning the workbook exercises the learner will want to become familiar with the following terms used in the chapter.

agnostic
atheist
faith
religion
spiritual beliefs
spiritual distress
spiritual needs
spirituality

Spirituality: True-False

Circle either the word True or the word False. If the statement is false, correct it in the space provided by changing the italicized words.

1. The spiritual dimension of the human person was recognized ***only since 2000 AD.***
   true false
   ____
2. The human person has been viewed as an integrated whole ***only since the holistic health movement.***
   true false
   ____
3. Nurses ***cannot*** assist clients to meet spiritual needs, but should ***always*** make a referral.
   true false
   ____
4. Persons who do not believe in God ***do not*** have spiritual needs.
   true false
   ____
5. Some religious beliefs are generally health-***denying and life-inhibiting.***
   true false
   ____
6. ***All Jewish infants*** are required to be circumcised on the 8th day after birth.
   true false
   ____
7. Protestant clients ***may request*** communion during illness.
   true false
   ____
8. ***Baptists and Disciples of Christ*** believe that baptism should not be administered until the person reaches the age of accountability.
   true false
   ____
9. The Friends denomination of Protestants ***reject*** both ordinances and sacraments.
   true false
   ____

10. Sacraments similar to those in the Catholic faith are *rejected by all* Protestant denominations.

    true false

    ____

Spirituality : Completion

Complete the sentences/phrases below by providing the missing word(s) in the blank spaces provided.

11. The doctrine of Jehovah's Witnesses prohibits ______________.
12. People of the Islamic faith believe that they are largely ______________ in controlling their fate.
13. Some people view illness as ______________ for ______________.
14. Some Navajo Indians believe ______________ will cure certain diseases.
15. There are 3 forms of Judaism, namely: ______________, ______________ and ______________.
16. ______________ form of Judaism is the most traditional and ______________ Judaism is the most liberal of the 3 forms.
17. Treatments and procedures should not be scheduled for observant Jewish clients on the __________ and ______________.
18. If desired by a dying Jewish client, a _______ should be called for ______________ and prayer.
19. The sacrament of ____________ for a Catholic client involves confession of sins.
20. ______________ is the most revered of all sacraments of the Catholic faith.

Spirituality: Matching

Match the letter preceding the factors which influence a person's spirituality with the numbered mini-personal situations below.

Factors:

A. Developmental considerations
B. Family
C. Ethnic Background
D. Formal Religion
E. Life Events

21. ____ A teenager and her parents are Islamic and read the Koran as scripture.
22. ____ Five year old Mary has prayed earnestly for a baby sister and firmly believes God can send her one.
23. ____ Robert's parents spend much time with him, play ball with him, take the family camping and share child care and housework. Robert believes God is just like his daddy.

24. ____ A farmer was very happy about his recent religious experience and prayed earnestly for rain during a drought. His crops were ruined by the drought and he stopped going to church.
25. ____ An African family came to the USA where the woman attempted to obtain her nursing degree. Her husband objected strongly when activities in nursing violated their beliefs and practices.

Spirituality : Matching

Draw a line from the type of spiritual distress (diagnosis) on the left to the behavior/statement on the right which demonstrates the specific diagnosis.

Diagnoses:	*Client Behavior:*
A. Spiritual anxiety	26."It seems unfair and makes me real mad at God that He let me get sick like this."
B. Spiritual despair	
C. Spiritual guilt	27. "I feel so isolated. It seems like God and my family are so far away."
D. Spiritual anger	28. "I guess God doesn't love me anymore. It seems He has turned His back on me just when I've lost everything."
E. Spiritual alienation	
F. Spiritual pain	29. "I know we are not supposed to worry but I'm afraid for the future that God won't take care of everything."
G. Spiritual loss	30. "I know I was wrong and I was at fault. I wonder if God will ever forgive what I did."

Crossword Puzzle

Across

3. Skeptic, denies God is knowable
5. The nonmaterial realm of being, soul
7. Any state of wellness/illness
8. A supernatural being, nonmaterial
9. Conviction of the truth
11. Emotional suffering caused by loss, sorrow
12. Pertaining to relationship with a higher power
18. A thing/belief of worth, to hold worthy

20. Pertaining to races and cultures
22. To be bereft of something valuable
26. Ire, rage, wrath, fury
28. A transgression
29. To be troubled or upset
30. Suffering due to injury or distress
31. An organized system of beliefs about a higher power

Down

1. To estrange or set against
2. The intellect or understanding
3. Denies the existence of God
4. Concern or give attention
6. Complete confidence in something for which there is no proof. Belief/trust in God
9. The physical substance of man
10. To pardon - to cease to resent
13. A spiritual advisor
14. Any deviation from wellness
15. Strong feeling of affection
16. Necessities
17. Harmony, tranquility
19. State of gladness, happiness or delight
21. A patient
23. The act of caring for
24. A basic unit in society
25. To feel at fault for misconduct
27. To beseech God

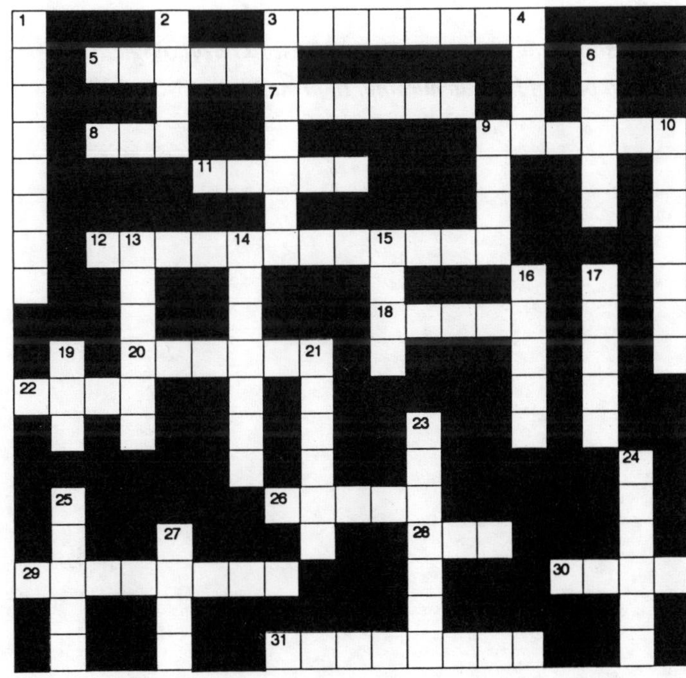

Additional Enrichment Activities

1. Attend one or more religious services in a denomination or religious group very different from those with which you are familiar. Make comparisons with your form of worship/religious experience. Evaluate what you liked/didn't like about the denomination you visited.
2. Initiate a conversation with a person from a different culture from yours and a faith different from yours (Christian if your are non-Christian or non-Christian if you are Christian). What do you have in common? What beliefs/practices are very different?

Suggested Readings

Clifford, M et al: Facilitating spiritual care in the rehabilitation setting. Rehabilitation Nursing 12(6):331-333, 1987

Ferszt, GG et al: When your patient needs spiritual comfort. Nursing 18(4):48-49, 1988

Forbis, PA: Meeting patients' spiritual needs: helping patients to fulfill their spiritual needs is part of the nursing process. Geriatric Nursing 9(3):158-159, 1988

Kennison, MM: Faith: an untapped health resource. J Psychosocial Nursing and Mental Health Services 25(10):28-30, 1987

Lane, JA: The care of the human spirit. J Professional Nursing 3(6):332-337, 1987

MacInnis K: Prayers. American J Nursing 87(9):1256, 1987

Mull, CS et al: Religion's role in the health and well-being of well elders. Public Health Nursing 4(3):151-159, 1987

O'Connor, PM: Spiritual elements of hospice care. Hospice 2(2):99-108, 1986

Reed, PG: Spirituality and well-being in terminally ill hospitalized adults. Research in Nursing and Health 10(5):335-344, 1987

Richter, JM: Support: a resource during crisis of mate loss. J Gerontological Nursing 13(11):18-22, 1987

Sims, C: Spiritual care as a part of holistic nursing. Imprint 34(4):63-64, 1987

Unit IX
Promoting Optimal Health in Special Situations

The four chapters comprising Unit IX of Taylor's Fundamentals of Nursing (1988) are concerned with the nurse's role in medication administration, diagnostic procedures, wound care, and care of the client having surgery.

Chapter 40
Medications

The nursing process is the organizing framework for Chapter 40, Medications (Taylor, 1988). Medication administration, a basic nursing function, is presented in order that the learner can approach this nursing function with the expected knowledge base.
After studying this chapter and completing the related workbook exercises, the learner should be able to

- Define key terms used in the chapter.
- Discuss drug legislation in the United States and Canada.
- Describe drug names, types of preparation, and types of drug orders.
- Identify drug classifications and actions.
- Discuss adverse effects of drugs, including allergy, tolerance, cumulative effect, idiosyncratic effect, and interactions.
- Obtain client information necessary to establish a medication history.
- Calculate drug dosages, using the various systems of equivalents.
- Describe principles used to safely prepare and administer medications, orally, parenterally, topically, and by inhalation.
- Develop teaching plans to meet client needs specific to medication administration.

Key Terms Chapter 40

The learner will find the workbook exercises most useful if, prior to attempting the activities, the definitions of the key terms have been mastered.

absorption
ampule
anaphylactic
antagonist effect
body surface area
bolus
chemical name
cumulative effect
diluent
distribution
drug
drug allergy
drug tolerance
excretion
generic name
heparin lock
iatrogenic disease
idiosyncratic effect
individual supply
inhalation
injections
instillation
intradermal
intramuscular
intravenous
inunction
irrigation
medication
medication order
metabolism
official name
parenteral
pharmacodynamics
pharmacokinetics
pharmacology
piggyback
prefilled cartridge
prescription
receptor
reconstitution
stock supply
subcutaneous
synergistic effect
topical application
trade name
unit dose
vial
Z-track

Key Terms: Match

Match the definitions on the left to the key terms on the right. Each term is used only once.

A. absorption
B. ampule
C. bolus
D. diluent
E. drug allergies
F. drug tolerance
G. drug interaction
H. idiosyncratic effect
I. intradermal
J. inunction
K. parenteral
L. pharmacokinetics
M. piggyback
N. trade name
O. vial
P. Z-track
Q. iatrogenic

1. ____ a glass bottle with a self sealing stopper through which medicine is removed
2. ____ a glass flask containing a single dose of medication
3. ____ the study of the movement of drug molecules
4. ____ the process by which a drug is transferred from its site of entry into the bloodstream
5. ____ an injection placed below the epidermis
6. ____ injection used to administer medications that are highly irritating to subcutaneous tissue
7. ____ drug administered by injection

8. ____ a medication mixed with a small amount of solution and given with the ongoing IV
9. ____ when a drug is incorporated in an agent and is rubbed into the skin for absorption
10. ____ a solution used to dilute a powder for injection
11. ____ a predetermined dose of medication given by IV push
12. ____ a disease caused unintentionally by drug therapy
13. ____ when the body becomes accustomed to drug over a period of time
14. ____ an abnormal or peculiar response to a drug that may manifest itself by an unexpected response
15. ____ combined effect of two or more drugs acting simultaneously producing either an effect less than or greater than each drug alone
16. ____ occurs in an individual who has been previously exposed to the drug and has developed antibodies
17. ____ name given to a drug by the company that developed the drug

Med Abbreviation Jeopardy

Let's play Jeopardy! Below are the answers. You supply the questions concerning each abbreviation.

18. OS What is the abbreviation for ____________________?
19. OD What is the abbreviation for ____________________?
20. OU What is the abbreviation for ____________________?
21. KVO What is the abbreviation for ____________________?
22. IVPB What is the abbreviation for ____________________?
23. DC What is the abbreviation for ____________________?
24. hs What is the abbreviation for ____________________?
25. IM What is the abbreviation for ____________________?
26. IV What is the abbreviation for ____________________?
27. pc What is the abbreviation for ____________________?
28. ac What is the abbreviation for ____________________?
29. ad lib What is the abbreviation for ____________________?
30. aq What is the abbreviation for ____________________?
31. ung What is the abbreviation for ____________________?
32. tid What is the abbreviation for ____________________?
33. supp What is the abbreviation for ____________________?
34. qd What is the abbreviation for ____________________?
35. qh What is the abbreviation for ____________________?
36. qid What is the abbreviation for ____________________?
37. qod What is the abbreviation for ____________________?
38. rx What is the abbreviation for ____________________?
39. SC What is the abbreviation for ____________________?
40. susp What is the abbreviation for ____________________?
41. aa What is the abbreviation for ____________________?
42. bid What is the abbreviation for ____________________?

43. $\bar{c}$ What is the abbreviation for ________________________?
44. cap What is the abbreviation for ________________________?
45. elix What is the abbreviation for ________________________?
46. PO What is the abbreviation for ________________________?
47. per What is the abbreviation for ________________________?
48. PRN What is the abbreviation for ________________________?
49. qs What is the abbreviation for ________________________?
50. stat What is the abbreviation for ________________________?
51. Tinct What is the abbreviation for ________________________?

Calculating Medication Dosages

In administering medications, you find a certain amount of the medication has been ordered by the physician and you have a different amount on hand. Make the necessary conversions and state what you will give to each patient.

52. Order: Gentamicin 60mg. On hand is Gentamicin 80 mg/2cc.
    Give: ___________
53. Order: aspirin gr V. On hand is aspirin 300mg/tab.
    Give: ___________
54. Order: Mestinon 30 mg. On hand is Mestinon 60 mg/tab.
    Give:___________
55. Order: amitriptyline 75 mg. On hand is amitriptyline 25mg/tab.
    Give: ___________
56. Order: phenylbutazone 250 mg. On hand is phenylbutazone 500mg/tab.
    Give: ___________
57. Order: ProBanthine 4 mg. On hand is ProBanthine 15 mg/tab.
    Give: ___________
58. Order: Penicillin V 125 mg. On hand is Penicillin V 500mg/tab.
    Give: ___________
59. Order: Lanoxin 0.125mg. On hand is Lanoxin 0.250 mg/tab.
    Give: ___________
60. Order: metaproterenol sulfate 20 mg. On hand is metaproterenol sulfate 10 mg/tab.
    Give: ___________
61. Order: ACTH 40 mg. On hand is ACTH 10 mg/cc.
    Give: ___________

Drug Preparations: Definitions

Define the following terms.

62. Capsule

____

63. Elixir

64. Liniment

65. Lotion

66. Lozenge

67. Ointment

68. Pill

69. Solution

70. Suppository

71. Suspension

72. Syrup

73. Tablet

Common Abbreviations for Measures

Provide the abbreviations for the following measures.

74. dram
75. drops
76. grain
77. milligram
78. milliliter
79. minim
80. ounce
81. tablespoon
82. teaspoon

Medication Procedures

Briefly explain how one performs the following drug administration procedures.

83. Heparin lock

84. IV piggyback

Additional Enrichment Activities

1. Contact your local pharmacist and interview him or her.
   A. Determine what kind of educational preparation is necessary to become a pharmacist.
   B. What are the legal boundaries of the profession?
   Is continuing education required for relicensure?
   C. What does he/she see as the nurses role in drug administration?
2. Accompany a nurse responsible for IV therapy. Observe especially for the following:
   A. Sterile/aseptic technique
   B. How the nurse starts and discontinues an IV
   C. How the nurse manages a "problem" IV and what is done when an IV becomes infiltrated
   D. Nurse-client interaction
3. Role play with your classmates
   A. How to prepare medications. Include the three safety checks.
   B. How to identify a patient prior to administering a medication.
   C. How to prepare a client for an injection in the dorsogluteal site.

Suggested Readings

Beaumont, E: IV infusion pumps. Nursing Management 18(9):26,28,30+, 1987

Cohen, MR: Always prepare an IV admixture before labelling the container. Nursing 18(3):10, 1988

Cohen, MR: Are errors waiting to happen? Nursing 18(9):18, 1988

Farley, D: How FDA approves new drugs. FDA Consumer 21(10):6-13, 1987

Fischer, RG: The meaning of FDA approval. Pediatric Nursing 13(5):360, 1987

Hanson, MJS: Hematoma associated with subcutaneous heparin administration. Focus on Critical Care 14(6):62-65, 1987

Manzo, M: A drug by any other name: your guide to brand and generic names. Nusing 18(3):96-107, 1988

Millema, SJ et al: Geriatric IV therapy. J Intravenous Nursing 11(1):56-61, 1988

Mockus, E: Making pain control easy...the button infuser. RN 51(3):82, 1988

Nieweg, R et al: A patient education program for a continuous infusion regimen on an outpatient basis. Cancer Nursing 10(4):177-182, 1987

Plastares S: Documentation of the side effects of medication. Home Health Care Nurse May/June 5(3):38-38, 1987Rodman, MJ: What to expect from the newest drugs. RN 51(3):59-64, 1988

Sheridan, M: Developing a tool for appraisal of nurses' knowledge regarding medications. J Continuing Education in Nursing 19(2):84-87, 1988

Swithers, CM: Tools for teaching about anticoagulants. RN 51(1):57-58, 1988

Tolbert, RB: Health professionals should monitor workers' over-the-counter drug use. Occupational Health and Safety 56(13):52, 54-55, 60, 1987

Westfall, LK et al: Why the elderly are so vulnerable to drug reactions. RN 50(11):39-43, 1987

Will surgery complicate your patient's drug therapy? Emergency Medicine 19(18):56-60,65,69-70+, 1987

Computer Assisted Instruction

Basic Math and Dosage Calculation. Mosbysystems.

Calculate with Care. JB Lippincott Company.

Drug Dosage, Calculations, and Administration. Medi-Sim, Inc.

Drug Dosage Review: Drill and Practice. Medi-Sim, Inc.

Drug Dosage Calculations: Practice Problems with Tutorial. Medi-Sim, Inc.

MedMath. JB Lippincott Company.

Pharmacology I, II, III, & IV. Medi-Sim, Inc.

Pharmacology CAI Series. Medi-Sim, Inc.

Chapter 41
Diagnostic Procedures

This chapter of Fundamentals of Nursing by Taylor (1988) introduces the learner to the responsibilities of the nurse in assisting with diagnostic tests. Included is content relevant to obtaining informed consent as well as preparing the client physically and psychologically.

After studying this chapter and completing the workbook activities the learner should be able to

- Define key terms used in the chapter.
- Describe various diagnostic tests and their purpose.
- Describe nursing responsibilities for a client prior to, during, and following a diagnostic test.
- Discuss the importance of psychologic preparation and support to clients having diagnostic tests.

Key Terms Chapter 41

Prior to attempting the workbook activities, the student is advised to study the key concepts associated with Chapter 41.

ascites
atrioventricular (AV) node
barium enema
biopsy
bronchoscopy
cholecystogram
computed tomography
colonoscopy
cystoscopy
depolarize
electrocardiogram
electrocardiograph
electroencephalogram
electroencephalograph
endoscope
endoscopic retrograde cholangiopancreatography
esophagogastroduodenoscopy
fasting state
fluoroscopy
intravenous pyelogram
leads
liver biopsy
lumbar puncture
magnetic resonance imaging (MRI)
paracentesis
polarity
proctosigmoidoscopy
Purkinje system
radiography
radioisotope
radiopaque
repolarize
sinoatrial (SA) node
spinal tap
thoracentesis
transducer
ultrasonography
ultrasound waves
upper gastrointestinal (GI)series
urinalysis
x-ray

Diagnostic Procedures: Paragraph Completion

Complete the following paragraphs related to nursing and diagnostic procedures.

1. Nursing responsibilities in relation to diagnostic procedures may include _______ _______ _______ as directed by the physician; _______ the test; preparing the client both _______ and _______ as well as providing for client _______ following the test; disposal of_________; and proper care of the _______.

2. It is important for the nurse to know the proper _______ when multiple exams are ordered. A _______ __________ must be scheduled _______ an _______ _____ because barium may interfere with _______ of the kidneys.

3. Following a _______ _________ the client is assisted to lie on the _______ side with a pillow or folded towel under the needle _______ _______. This position must be maintained for several hours to prevent the complication of _______.

4. The nurse may be requested to assist with the _______ test performed during a lumbar puncture. While the needle is in the subarachnoid space, pressure is applied to the

client's _______ _______. An _______ in CNS pressure is a _______response. A _______ in the spinal fluid will _______ the pressure from _______.

5. The client undergoing a thoracentesis must be assessed _______ and _______ the procedure. The client's _______,_______, and _______ are carefully monitored. _______, _______, and _______ can occur during the procedure. Following the procedure, _______ _________ may become acute if the lung has been accidentally __________________. The physician should be promptly notified if the client has _______ _______ or _______ sputum.

6. The _______ is a valuable tool that aids in the diagnosis of conditions such as _______ or _______ diseases. The client needs a clear understanding that the procedure does _______ cause any _______ or _______ even though electrodes are attached to the _________. Another use for this test is to determine _______ _______.

Diagnostic Exam: Matching

Match the following diagnostic examinations with their definitions. (Some terms may be used more than once).

Terms:

A. computed tomography
B. electrocardiogram
C. electroencephalogram
D. endoscopy
E. liver biopsy
F. lumbar puncture
G. Magnetic Resonance Imaging (MRI)
H. paracentesis
I. radioisotope scanning
J. thoracentesis
K. ultrasonography

Definitions:

7. _____ its use is helpful in obtaining tissue samples for examination
8. _____ withdrawal of fluid from subarachnoid space
9. _____ produces a cross-sectional image of a body part
10. _____ involves aspiration of fluid from the pleural cavity
11. _____ recording of the electrical impulses of the heart
12. _____ recording of the pattern of sound waves as reflected off body tissues
13. _____ uses magnetism and radiowaves to produce cross-sectional images of body tissues
14. _____ removal of a tiny amount of liver tissue
15. _____ used to measure pressure of the cerebrospinal fluid
16. _____ recording of the electrical impulses of the brain
17. _____ involves aspiration of fluid from peritoneal cavity

18. _____ requires intake or ingestion of a radioisotope which localizes in a target organ
19. _____ allows direct visualization of an organ or cavity
20. _____ while electrodes are attached to the chest and extremities this test causes no sensation or discomfort
21. _____ a common name for this test is CT-scan
22. _____ procedure done to alleviate ascites

Nursing Interventions: Timeframe

Select the correct time parameter for the nursing actions listed below. In some cases an action may require more than one answer.

A - Pre test preparation
B - During the test or procedure
C - Following the examination

23. _____ send appropriately labeled specimens to the laboratory
24. _____ clarify with the physician which medications may be given and which must be held
25. _____ record client reactions on the bedside flowsheet
26. _____ assist the client in maintaining a prescribed position
27. _____ assess physical and emotional response
28. _____ provide warmth, pain relief and provide explanations
29. _____ schedule the procedure with the appropriate department
30. _____ place necessary equipment in the client's room or examination room
31. _____ provide additional supplies and maintain sterility
32. _____ administer the ordered sedative medication
33. _____ encourage client to verbalize fears and concerns
34. _____ monitor for adverse reactions such as respiratory distress or hemorrhage

Diagnostic Test Identification

Identify (name) each of the following diagnostic procedures.

35. Visual examination of the entire large intestine:

____

36. Visual examination of the trachea and bronchi:

____

37. Visual examination of the large intestine by use of a radiopaque medium:

____

38. X-ray visualization of the gallbladder:

____

39. Visual examination of the esophagus, stomach and duodenum:

____

40. Visualization of the kidney's ability to excrete urine:

41. Visual examination of the bladder, urethra, and ureteral orifices:

42. Visual examination of the stomach and small intestines by use of a radiopaque medium:

43. Visual examination of the rectum, rectosigmoid junction, and lower sigmoid colon:

44. A blood sugar test which is collected at a time when the client has been abstaining from food or fluids:

Diagnostic Tests Commonalities

Can you identify what these tests have in common? Answers may pertain to preparation of the client, performance of the exam or procedures following the examination.

45. Upper GI series and barium enema:

46. Electrocardiogram and electroencephalogram:

47. Thoracentesis and paracentesis:

48. Upper GI and gastroscopy:

49. Liver biopsy and lumbar puncture:

50. Liver sonogram and routine urinalysis:

Nursing Diagnoses

Write at least three nursing diagnoses that would apply to the client having a diagnostic test.

51.
52.
53.

Additional Enrichment Activities

1. If possible, visit each of the following departments: Medical Laboratory, Radiology, Nuclear Medicine, Endoscopy Laboratory, EKG Laboratory, EEG Laboratory
2. Which tests are performed by each of these departments? What do clients experience with these tests?
3. How do personnel relate to clients? To the nurses on your nursing unit?
4. Assist or observe the preparation of a client for an x-ray examination; an EKG; and EEG; an endoscopy procedure; a blood or urine test; and a nuclear medicine treatment or test. How does client preparation compare or differ from each of these examinations?
5. Interview clients on the nursing unit where you are assigned for clinical. Ask them about their preparations for their exams or procedures. Did they feel they were well prepared and knowledgeable or do they have suggestions for ways they could have been better prepared or less anxious.
6. Scan client charts to determine how diagnostic test preparation, administration and reporting are documented. Are all three phases consistently documented? Can you identify abnormal test results?

Suggested Readings

Caine, R: Essentials of monitoring the electrocardiogram. Nursing Clinics of North America 22(1):77-87, 1987

Collins, M: The dreaded Mrs. Scott...never "assume" a patient was malingering. AD Nurse 2(3):18-19, 1987

Crowell, M et al: Implementation of electrocardiographic monitoring in labor and delivery. Focus on Critical Care 15(1):19-22, 1988

Findlay, S: Are we hooked on tests? US News and World Report 103(21):60-65, 1987

Fischback FT: Manual of laboratory diagnostic tests. 3rd Ed. JB Lippincott Company, 1988

Fredette, SL: Common diagnostic errors. Nurse Educator 13(3):31-36, 1988

Henrietta, G: Lab tests you can't overlook...certain drugs can cause physiologic problems. Nursing 17(2):56-59, 1987

Johnston, JB: Laboratory tests: clinical, financial, and professional implications. Emergency Nursing Reports 2(10):1-8, 1988

Larson, JL et al: Computerized arrhythmia monitoring. J Cardiovascular Nursing 2(1):58-66, 1987

Lunney, M et al: Educating nurse diagnosticians. Nurse Educator 13(1):24-29, 1988

Parker, BM: Electrocardiography: identifying diagnostic pitfalls. Consultant 27(8):34-38, 1987

Powills, S: New imaging tool developed by researchers. Hospitals 61(20):75, 1987

Tanner, CA et al: Diagnostic reasoning strategies of nurses and nursing students. Nursing Research 36(6):358-363, 1987

Witkin, GB et al: Choosing liver function tests. Emergency Medicine 19(20):22-26, 1987

Zelus, PR et al: Dialing for health: electrocardiogram analysis program. Geriatric Nursing 9(4):230-231, 1988

Evaluating the usefulness of routine preoperative tests. AORN J 45(3):696, 1987

Chapter 42
Care of Wounds

Chapter 42 of the Fundamentals of Nursing text (Taylor, 1988) provides the student with opportunity to gain knowledge about wounds, wound healing, and wound care. The use of the nursing process, including selected nursing diagnoses for the client with a wound, is presented in the text. The following workbook exercises provide additional learning opportunities for the student to apply nursing process in the care of the clients with a several types of wounds.

After completing this chapter and the workbook exercises, the learner should be able to

- Define key terms used in the chapter.
- Describe the physical and psychologic effects of trauma to the body, with resultant wounds.
- Discuss the processes involved in wound healing.
- Describe wound complications, integrating factors affecting wound healing.
- Summarize emergency wound assessment and care.
- Describe the effects of the application of heat or cold.
- Use the nursing process to knowledgeably derive an individualized plan of care for the client with a wound, including the application of dressings and heat or cold.

Key Terms Chapter 42

Prior to attempting the workbook exercises, the learner will want to become familiar with the following key terms used in Chapter 42.

abrasion
abscess
bandage
binder
capillarity
closed wound
compress
contusion
dehiscence
dressing
evisceration
exudate
granulation tissue
incision
laceration
many-tailed binder
open wound
pack
puncture
purulent
retention sutures
sanguineous
scar
scultetus binder
serous
sitz bath
skin sutures
stab wound
wound

Wound Types

Read the following descriptions and select the appropriate type of wound for each description in both sets.

A - Intentional wound
B - Unintentional wound

1. ____ jagged wound edges
2. ____ high risk for infection
3. ____ bleeding controlled
4. ____ multiple tissue trauma
5. ____ planned therapy
6. ____ sterile supplies utilized
7. ____ healing facilitated
8. ____ gunshot wound

A - Open wound
B - Closed wound

9. ____ internal injury and hemorrhaging may occur
10. ____ skin is not broken
11. ____ may be intentional or unintentional
12. ____ usually unintentional
13. ____ increased risk of infection
14. ____ some bleeding may occur
15. ____ injuries from strain or fall
16. ____ cut or laceration

Wound Descriptors

Complete the short paragraphs regarding wound descriptors.

17. A bruise or ________ is caused by a blow from a ________ object. It is a ________ wound which results in soft-tissue damage and ruptured ________ ________. ________ and ________ are symptoms of this type of wound. Serious effects may result if________ ________ are contused.

18. A surgical incision is also an ________ wound. Incisions are performed under surgical ________, with a sharp ________ or ________.
19. A ________ wound is made by a sharp instrument that ________ the ____ and underlying ________. Puncture wounds may be either ________ or unintentional.
20. A wound with torn, __________ edges is described as a ________. It is usually due to accidental ________. When caused by an ________ object there is a greater risk of ________.
21. A painful, open wound which involves only the skin is called an ________. They may result from either an accidental _______ or from ________ dermatological procedures.

Wound Characteristics: Matching

Match the following:

22. ____ increased risk of infection
23. ____ closed wound
24. ____ purulent drainage
25. ____ high risk of infection
26. ____ surgical incision
27. ____ GI surgery
28. ____ inflamed wound
29. ____ break in asepsis
30. ____ old, traumatic wound
31. ____ no pathogenic organisms

Characteristics:

A. Clean
B. Clean-contaminated
C. Contaminated
D. Infected

Word Scramble

Complete the blanks with the appropriate key term. Then locate each word in the "word scramble." Words may be located vertically, diagonally, horizontally or backwards.

32. ______________________________ of wound edges enhances healing
33. A lasticized material makes a good ________________________
34. A ______________________________ offers support for a wound
35. ______________________________ produces vasoconstriction
36. A bruise is also called a ______________________________
37. Wet to dry dressings are used for wound ____________________
38. A protective covering is called a ________________________
39. ________________________ to dry dressings may be used to debride wounds
40. ________________________ occurs when the viscera protrudes through incision
41. Wound drainage is called ______________________________
42. New tissue is called ______________________________ tissue

43. ______________________ produces vasodilation
44. A ______________________ wound will produce swelling
45. An ____________________ is an intentional wound
46. A pack is usually hot and ______________________
47. A ______________________ is applied to an extensive body surface
48. A _____________________ penetrates the skin
49 ______________________ drainage contains white blood cells
50. ______________________ ____________ offer added support to incision
51 Red ____________________ drainage indicates bleeding
52. A healed incision is called a ______________________
53. A many-tailed binder is also called a ______________ ______________
54. Clear ____________________ portion of the blood is a type of drainage
55. ______________________ sutures are usually made of silk
56. A ____________________ ____________ is a separate drain opening
57. Many wounds occur from ______________________
58. Wet to____________________ dressings are used for debridement
59. Any skin opening is called a ______________________

```
CHEMORRHAGICIFMT
USCULTETUSBINDER
DCPOGKTFQARDCBMA
ERGDLDEOTBNAIXOU
BERRDDNSHUKFSAIM
RVAEEFTGOMZCIWSA
IINSHQIWEPANOBTX
DSUSILOKXRGHNPMA
ECLISANGUINEOUSZ
MEANCFSVDQDASNEI
ERTGERUIAGNTNCRT
NAIANATBTCFOVTOM
TTOLCHUIEZIJKUUU
BINDERRSQSKINRSL
VOWARTERUPONLEMA
XNBKCYSTABWOUNDZ
EHCFBANDAGEGHIMO
VAPPROXIMATIONJR
PXFMCVQPURULENTQ
```

Surgical Drains

Identify (name) each of the following types of drains:

60. Collects drainage to decrease dead space. Used after breast removal or abdominal surgery: ________
61. Used for infected wounds or hemorrhoid surgery. Allows healing from base of wound: ________
62. Provides a sinus tract for drainage following abdominal surgery or to drain an abscess: ________
63. Decreases dead space by collecting drainage. Used after orthopedic or abdominal surgery: ________
64. Used following gallbladder surgery for the drainage of bile: ________

Wound Care: True/False

Select either ***true*** or ***false*** for the following statements. Correct the false statements.

65. Betadine, 70% alcohol, 3% hydrogen peroxide, and sterile normal saline are commonly antiseptic cleansing agents
    true ***false*** ________
66. Acetate tape is used primarily for compression or pressure dressings.
    true ***false*** ________
67. Phase I healing occurs from the time of the incision to the second day following surgery.
    true ***false*** ________
68. Increased urinary output and a decreased hemoglobin may be signs of wound hemorrhage.
    true ***false*** ________
69. Pins, knots or seams in a bandage or binder can cause great discomfort for the client.
    true ***false*** ________
70. The frequency of dressing changes depends on the amount of drainage, physician preference and nature of the wound.
    true ***false*** ________
71. The nurse documents assessments and interventions regarding wound care on a daily basis.
    true ***false*** ________
72. Montgomery straps require changing with each dressing as do regular tape strips.
    true ***false*** ________
73. When removing sutures (or staples), every other suture should be removed first to be sure the wound is healed.
    true ***false*** ________

74. "Teach client the importance of protein in promoting wound healing" would be an appropriate nursing intervention for the goal of: "client will participate in self-care activities promoting wound healing".
true false ______________________

Nursing Actions in Wound Care

Provide the rationale for the following nursing actions.

75. Apply aquathermia pad or external heating device over sterile compress to an open wound.
____
____

76. Fill hot water bag 1/2 to 2/3 full and expel remaining air.
____
____

77. When collecting a wound culture, carefully insert swab into drainage and roll gently.
____
____

78. When irrigating a wound, try to maintain a steady flow of solution and continue irrigation until solution returns clear.
____
____

79. When cleaning a wound, clean from top to bottom or from center outwardly.
____
____

Nursing Diagnoses/Interventions

List at least three possible nursing interventions for each of the following nursing diagnoses related to wounds.

80. Knowledge deficit regarding wound care and dressing changes at home
   A. ______________________
   B. ______________________
   C. ______________________
81. Potential for infection related to purulent wound drainage
   A. ______________________
   B. ______________________
   C. ______________________

82. Alteration in comfort: pain related to abdominal incision
   A. ______________________________
   B. ______________________________
   C. ______________________________

Additional Enrichment Activities

1. Phone local pharmacies, medical supply distributors, etc. to locate availability of disposable wound care supplies in your area.
2. From the above resources, make an estimate of the cost to the client for two dressing changes per day including the following supplies:
   a. 4 ABD's (or surgipads) sterile
   b. 8 packages of sterile 4x4's
   c. alcohol (one bottle)
   d. cotton tipped applicators (4 packages of 2 each)
   e. Betadine swabs (3 packages of 3 each)
   f. 2 large telfa dressings
   g. sterile gloves (at least one pair)
3. What would be the approximate cost to the client for one week?
4. Make a visit with a home health care nurse to a client's home who requires wound care and/or dressing changes. Observe not only the dressing change procedures, but also the nurse's role and the client's needs/reactions.
5. In clinical, observe or assist an RN with the following procedures: dressing change, wound culture, wound irrigation, application of hot or cold treatment. Observe not only the procedure, but the client's needs/reactions.
6. Try to identify clients who may be at risk for the development of wound complications (for example, individuals who are very old or malnourished). What could you as the nurse do to decrease their risk?

Suggested Readings

Fay MF: Drainage systems: their role in wound healing AORN 46(3):442-443, 445, 447+, 1988

Lamb C: Suiting the dressing to the wound. Patient Care 21(11):164-166, 169, 173+, 1987

Mather DG, et al: A form that makes wound assessment easier. RN 50(6):37-39, 1987

Neuberger GB et al: Wound care: what's clear, what's not. Nursing 17(2):34-37, 1987

Serggreen MY: Healing of physical wounds. Nursing Clinics of North America 22(2):439-447, 1987

Chapter 43
Perioperative Care

Chapter 43 of Fundamentals of Nursing, (Taylor, 1988) discusses the nursing care appropriate during the three phases of the perioperative period.
After studying the chapter and completing the workbook exercises, the learner should be able to

- Define key terms used in the chapter.
- Describe the surgical experience; including perioperative phases, categories of surgery, types of anesthesia, and informed consent.
- Conduct a preoperative nursing history and nursing examination to identify client strengths as well as factors increasing surgical and postoperative complication risk.
- Demonstrate preoperative exercises: deep-breathing, coughing, and leg exercises.
- Prepare a client physically and psychologically for surgery.
- Describe the nurse's role in the intraoperative phase.
- Identify assessments specific to the prevention of complications, promote a return to health, and facilitate coping with alterations.
- Plan and implement interventions for ongoing postoperative care to prevent complications, promote a return to health, and facilitate coping with alterations.
- Use the nursing process to knowledgeably develop an individualized plan of care for the surgical client during each phase of the perioperative period.

Key Terms Chapter 43

Prior to attempting the workbook exercises, the learner will want to become familiar with the following key terms used in Chapter 43.

ambulatory surgery
atelectasis
circulating nurse
dehiscence
elective surgery
emergency surgery
evisceration
general anesthesia
hemorrhage
holding area
hypovolemic shock
informed consent
intraoperative phase
paralytic ileus
perioperative period
pneumonia
postanesthesia recovery room
postoperative phase
preoperative phase
pulmonary embolus
regional anesthesia
scrub nurse
shock
thrombophlebitis

Surgery Classification

From the descriptions below, select the appropriate surgery classification. Complete all three sets.

Set A

1. ____ performed to preserve life
2. ____ coronary artery by-pass
3. ____ intestinal obstruction
4. ____ performed to improve self-concept
5. ____ performed to restore function
6. ____ mammoplasty

A. Urgent
B. Elective
C. Emergency

Set B

7. ____ may be either elective or emergency
8. ____ abdominal hysterectomy
9. ____ cataract extraction
10. ____ to remove a body part
11. ____ to correct deformities

A. Major
B. Minor

Set C

12. ____ performed to replace organs
13. ____ debridement of necrotic tissue
14. ____ restores function in congenital anomalies
15. ____ bronchoscopy
16. ____ to improve self-concept
17. ____ colon resection
18. ____ is not a curative surgery
19. ____ skin graft for burns
20. ____ to make or confirm a diagnosis
21. ____ cleft palate repair

A. Diagnostic
B. Ablative
C. Palliative
D. Reconstructive
E. Transplant
F. Constructive

Levels of Anesthesia

List the client feelings experienced in each stage of general anesthesia and state the level of consciousness for each.

22. Stage 1: ____

23. Stage 2: ____

24. Stage 3: ____

25. Stage 4: ____

Local and Regional Anesthesia

Differentiate between the following types of local or regional anesthetics. Include location of anesthesia, uses, and major side effects if given in text.

Type of anesthesia	Location	Uses	Side Effects
26. Subdural block:			
27. Topical:			
28. Nerve block:			
29. Local infiltration:			

Perioperative True/False

Select True or False for the following statements regarding perioperative nursing (explain why false statements are false).

30. Clients agree to surgery by verbal consent.
    true false ____

31. Ambulatory surgery is provided on an outpatient basis; preoperative teaching is usually unnecessary.
    true false ______________________________
32. Surgical procedures are categorized by urgency, risk and purpose.
    true false ______________________________
33. Preoperative assessment is aimed at the identification of physical risk factors.
    true false ______________________________
34. Surgery is a stressful time for both the client and family, imposing physical and psychosocial alterations and adaptations.
    true false ______________________________
35. Intraoperative nursing roles are either as a scrub nurse or a circulating nurse.
    true false ______________________________
36. The nursing process is used throughout the perioperative period to provide knowledgeable, holistic, individualized care.
    true false ______________________________
37. Ambulatory surgery can usually still be performed even if the client has a cold or infection.
    true false ______________________________
38. Client teaching regarding the surgery is done during the immediate postoperative period.
    true false ______________________________
39. Ongoing postoperative care includes the client and family and is planned to facilitate recovery from surgery.
    true false ______________________________

Client Goals

Write an appropriate client goal for each of the following nursing diagnoses.

A. Preoperative nursing diagnoses:

40. Knowledge deficit: Preoperative surgical events

    ____
41. Knowledge deficit: postoperative exercises and activities

    ____

B. Intraoperative nursing diagnoses:

42. Potential for ineffective breathing pattern related to surgical position

    ____
43. Potential complication of surgery: nosocomial infection

    ____

C. Postoperative nursing diagnoses:

44. Potential alteration in respiratory function related to anesthesia and incisional pain

    ____
45. Potential fluid volume deficit related to excessive fluid loss from nasogastric suction and wound

    ____

46. Alteration in comfort: Acute pain related to abdominal incision

____

47. Knowledge deficit: discharge teaching for self care of surgical incision.

____

Postoperative Complications

The following terms refer to possible complications that could occur during or following surgery. Unscramble the terms and define the complication.

48. *Birhoteishmotbpl*

____

49. *Maponiuen*

____

50. *Regrnmroha*

____

51. *Ohskc*

____

52. *Tsaleisaetc*

____

53. *Aacpltiyr ulise*

____

54. *Ulmrapony Elmobsu*

____

55. *Tsavicnoerie*

____

Drugs and Surgical Risks

Surgical risk is increased by some drugs. Identify the drugs that can cause the following reactions:

56. May increase the hypotensive action of anesthetics:______________

57. May precipitate hemorrhage during or after surgery:______________

58. If abruptly withdrawn, client may suffer cardiovascular collapse:__________

59. Can cause respiratory paralysis when combined with certain muscle relaxants used during surgery:______________

60. May result in electrolyte imbalance and respiratory depression:__________

Nursing Interventions: Matching

Match the nursing intervention with the type of complication for which it was planned to monitor or prevent (an answer may be used more than once).

Interventions:

61. ____ Implement deep-breathing and coughing exercises
62. ____ Encourage ambulation
63. ____ Maintain a clean environment
64. ____ Implement leg exercises
65. ____ Use medical asepsis
66. ____ Assess for dehydration
67. ____ Encourage high fiber foods
68. ____ Assess and record Homan's sign
69. ____ Position to increase ventilation
70. ____ Maintain IV fluid intake
71. ____ Provide oral hygiene

Complications:

A. Cardiovascular
B. Respiratory
C. Elimination
D. Fluid & Electrolyte
E. Comfort
F. Wound

Rationale for Nursing Actions

State the rationale for the following nursing actions that pertain to perioperative care.

72. Promote optimum nutritional and hydration status.

    ____

73. Conduct preoperative teaching regarding coughing and deep breathing exercises, leg exercises and pain control.

    ____

74. Shave and prepare the operative site.

    ____

75. Have client empty bladder and bowel prior to surgery.

    ____

76. When performing a shave prep, report any cuts in skin to the physician or surgical charge nurse.

    ____

77. Provide warmth to client postoperatively.

    ____

78. Check dressings for drainage and feel under client for bleeding.

    ____

79. Turn client at least every 2 hours until client is able to turn by self.

    ____

80. Assess bowel sounds for return of peristalsis.

81. Monitor extremities for presence of edema.

82. Report adventitious lung sounds immediately.

83. Take vital signs prior to surgery.

Surgical Risk in the Elderly

List at least 2 changes in each system that result in surgery being a greater threat for the elderly client.

84. Renal:

85. Respiratory:

86. Cardiovascular:

87. Integument:

88. Neurologic:

Additional Enrichment Activities

1. In your clinical agency, assist or observe the nurse in preparation of clients having surgery with both a general anesthetic and local anesthetic. Compare and contrast the differences in preparation. Note the completion of a pre-operative check list.
2. If possible, spend a day in each of the following surgical departments: surgical holding area, operating room and recovery room. Observe both the functions performed by the nurse and the nurse-client interactions.
3. Observe both a surgery performed under general anesthesia and local anesthesia. See if you can identify the stages of anesthesia. Do personnel behave differently when the client is awake during the surgery as opposed to when the client is asleep?

4. Visit an out-patient free-standing surgical center and observe the entire perioperative process. Follow a client from admission to discharge and note when and what kind of teaching is done by the nurse.
5. On your clinical unit, try to identify clients who may be at risk for the development of surgical complications, ie: elderly persons, respiratory or cardiovascular clients.
6. Assist with or observe in the pre-operative teaching of a client to include: deep breathing and coughing exercises, leg exercises; incentive spirometer; pain control; and surgical expectations. Visit with the same client postoperatively and assess your preoperative teaching. Did the client feel prepared? Is he/she following instructions as taught?

Suggested Readings

Recommended practices: documentation of perioperative nursing care. AORN J 45(3):777, 779, 781, 1987

The integrated approach to the management of pain. NIH Consensus Development Conference J Pain Symptom Management 2(1):35-44, 1987

Appendix: Answers

Unit I: The Nurse: Foundations for Nursing Practice

Chapter 1: Introduction to Nursing

1-5. Contributions of Florence Nightingale
- a. Nutrition recognized as a part of nursing care.
- b. Nursing separate and distinct from medicine.
- c. Importance of continuing education for nurses.
- d. Instituted occupational and recreational therapy for the sick.
- e. Role of the nurse in identifying and meeting the personal needs of the patient.
- f. Establishing standard for hospital management.
- g. Establishing a respected occupation for women.
- h. Establishing nursing education, recognizing the two components of nursing: health and illness.

6. Miss Nightingale's contributions were remarkable for the period in which she lived because she was a woman in an era in which women in general, and nurses in particular, held relatively low social positions.

History of Nursing
7. deaconesses
8. 1820
9. apprenticeship

The Art of Nursing
10. Nursing is the demonstration of nonpossessive **caring** for and about others.
11. Nursing is **sharing** self with patients, other health-team members, and with each other.
12. Nursing is **touching** to provide comfort and give care.
13. Nursing is sharing with clients in the human **feelings** of sorrow, joy, frustration, and satisfaction.
14. Nursing is **listening** attentively to the verbal and nonverbal communication signals.
15. Nursing is **accepting** of self in order to accept others.
16. Nursing is **respecting** of individual differences through unconditional acceptance, ensuring confidences and privacy, and individualizing care.

Key Terms: Match
17. F
18. L
19. K
20. J
21. E
22. C
23. A
24. I
25. G
26. B
27. H
28. D

Crossword Puzzle

Down
1. laws
2. need
4. Montag
5. change
6. implement
8. education
9. LPN
11. continuum
13. ANA
15. nurse
17. diagnose
19. NLN
21. diploma
22. process
25. client

Across
3. assessment
7. health
10. autonomy
12. action
14. five
15. Nightengale
16. elderly
18. CNA
20. ICN
23. coping
24. NCLEX
26. NLN
28. masters
29. nursing
30. standards

Nursing Organization Acronyms
29. ANA: American Nurses' Association
30. ICN: International Council of Nurses
31. NLN: National League for Nursing
32. NSNA: National Student Nurses' Association
33. CNA: Canadian Nurses' Association

Expanded Nursing Roles
34. Nurse Midwife: a. certificate or advanced degree; provides pre & postnatal care & delivers babies in uncomplicated pregnancies

35. Nurse Practitioner: b. advanced degree, certified for a specialty area; works in a variety of settings providing health assessment & primary care
36. Nurse Anesthetist: c. advanced degree/certificate; administers & monitors anesthesia

Chapter 2: Promoting Wellness in Health and Illness

Factors Influencing Health-Illness

1. a) emotional, b) environmental, c) spiritual, d) intellectual, e) sociocultural, f) physical
2. a) experience of symptoms, b) dependent role, c) recovery & rehabilitation
3.

Health Good Normal Illness Death

←——————————→

4. Compare your response to the examples given in Fundamentals of Nursing (Taylor, 1988, p. 20).
5. 1st Diseases of the heart and blood vessels
   2nd Cancer
   3rd Accidents
   4th Chronic respiratory diseases
   5th Pneumonia & influenza
6. a) genetic defects, b) biologic toxins or agents, c) physical agents, d) developmental defects, e) hormone/enzyme imbalance, f) tissue response to injury or irritation, g) reaction to stress
7. a) common cold, b) pneumonia, c) appendicitis, d) flu
8. a) diabetes, b) multiple sclerosis, c) chronic kidney failure, d) arthritis

Health-Illness Key Terms Match

9. P
10. F
11. I
12. C
13. L
14. E
15. J
16. B
17. F
18. N
19. D
20. O
21. M
22. A
23. K

Level of Preventive Care

Primary:

28. Immunizations
29. Accident prevention
30. Dental care teaching

Secondary:

24. Giving meds
26. Decubitus care
27. Teaching self-breast exam
31. Physical therapy
32. ROM

Tertiary:

25. Facilitating a suporrt group
26. Diabetic instruction
33. *Case Study*

Level 1 - Physiological needs: control bleeding; safety of Joan and her fetus

Level 2 - Safety and security needs: security as pertains to welfare of her unborn child and family; financial concerns for family

Level 3 - Love and belonging needs: recent loss of spouse; fear, sadness, potential for a second loss of a loved one

Level 4 - Self-esteem needs: concern about what she might have done to influence this recent threat to her unborn child; questions about ability to cope with all the stressors and ability to provide for family

Level 5 -Self-actualization: while not a high priority interventions need to be carried out in an atmosphere that reaffirms Joan's worth

Chapter 3: The Health-Care System

Health-Care System: Match

1. A
2. B
3. D
4. C
5. E
6. B
7. C
8. D
9. A
10. E
11. D
12. C
13. A
14. B
15. B
16. C
17. A
18. E
19. D

Crossword Puzzle

Down	*Across*
2 PHS	1. hospice
3. HMO	4. MASH
5. AA	7. PPA
6. HHC	10. non-profit
7. public	12. client
8. DO	13. ADL
9. LTC	15. Medicare
10. nurses	16. DRG's
11. Red Cross	18. PPOs
14. RD	21. NIH
15. Medicaid	23. respite
17. SPU	26. waste
18. four	29. resolve
20. RT	30. MD
24. stroke	
25. OT	
27. ECG	
28. xray	

Health-Care System: Short Answer

20. a) encourage client to obtain all medication prescriptions from a single pharmacy; b) encourage client to communicate changes in treatment plans to each physician to keep them updated on care received by others; c) serve as client advocate and care coordinator in the hospital and community; d) promote the integration of inpatient and outpatient records when serving on agency policy committees.
21. A third party, the insurance company, pays the bills.
22. When pain relief, symptom management, and supportive services are requested/needed by a terminally ill client and his family.
23. a) independent living, b) community care, c) skilled inpatient nursing care
24. The Canadian health-care system is administered through health plans within each province which are financed by federal and provincial taxes. These plans cover all Canadian residents for most of their necessary hospital care and physician's fees. In the US there is a combination of federal, state, and city support for state and federal health care systems such as the VA, county/city hospitals, etc. State and national taxes aid in financing national health and welfare programs such as Medicare, Medicaid. All residents in the US are not covered by government health programs.

Health-Care Agency Completion

25. 1983, diagnostic related groups (DRGs)
26. voluntary agencies

Health-Care Team

27. Pharmacist; formulate and dispense medicines; college degree (4-6yrs); license
28. Physical Therapist; restore function or prevent disability; college degree (4 yrs); PT State License
29. Physicians' Assistant; responsibilities depend upon the physician supervising the activities; specific courses, certificate; PA title
30. Occupational Therapist; assist the physically challenged individual adapt to limitations; college degree (4 yrs); OT state license
31. Dietitian: responsible for managing and planning for the dietary needs of clients; college degree and/or internship; RD registration examination
32. Respiratory Therapist: administer techniques that will improve pulmonary function and oxygenation; specific courses, certificate or associate degree--varies; RT title

Chapter 4: Theoretical Base for Nursing Practice

Nursing Theory: Matching

1. H
2. F
3. I
4. B
5. E
6. A
7. C
8. L
9. M
10. J
11. N
12. K
13. D
14. G

Nursing Theory: Completion

15. a) person; b) health; c) environment; d) nursing
16. a. conceptual models and practice philosophy
    b. theories borrowed from other disciplines
    c. development of theory within the profession
17. Nursing Research; 1950
18. a. the internal (self)
    b. the social (others)
    c. the physical (biochemical reactions)
19. a. identifies and defines interrelated concepts
    b. must be simple and general
    c. must be logical in nature
    d. should increase nursing's body of knowledge
    e. should guide and improve practice

Theoretical Model: True/False

20. False
21. False
22. False

23. True
24. True
25. False

Chapter 5: Values and Ethics in Nursing

Values and Ethics: Matching

1. N
2. M
3. D
4. F
5. J
6. A
7. B
8. H
9. C
10. E
11. R
12. I
13. G
14. L

Value/Ethics: True/False

15. False
16. True
17. False
18. False
19. False
20. False
21. True

Values Clarification and Ethics: Completion

22. a. theoretical orientation
    b. economic orientation
    c. aesthetic orientation
    d. social orientation
    e. political orientation
    f. religious orientation
23. a. modeling
    b. moralizing
    c. laissez-faire
    d. rewarding and punishing
    e. responsible choice
24. a. choosing
    b. prizing
    c. acting
25. *Chooses* a) freely; b) from alternatives; c) after careful consideration of the consequences of each of the alternatives
    Prizes d) with pride and happiness; e) with public affirmation
    Acts (f) with incorporation of the choice into one's behavior; (g) with consistency and regularity on the value
26. a) altruism, b) equality, c) aesthetics, d) freedom, e) human dignity, f) justice, g) truth
27. Your explanation of professional ethical conduct should include elements of sources of moral authority, nursing code of ethics, and the patient's bill of rights.
28. Polarized models of decision making that place absolute authority for decisions in the hands of either the client or the physician are rejected in favor of a model that emphasizes mutual participation, respect, and shared decision-making.

29.-36. Case Study

Chapter 6: Legal Implications of Nursing

Legal Implications of Nursing: Match

1. E
2. F
3. V
4. A
5. K
6. Z
7. L
8. X
9. W
10. R
11. D
12. H
13. Q
14. U
15. O
16. J
17. B
18. G
19. M
20. N
21. P
22. Y
23. S
24. C
25. I
26. T

Legal Aspects of Nursing: True/False

27. True
28. True
29. True
30. False
31. False
32. False
33. True
34. True

Short Answer

35. a) constitutions; b) statutes; c) administrative law; d) common law
36. a) unprofessional conduct; b) fraud; c) deceptive practices, d) criminal acts; e) previous discipli-

nary action by other state boards; f) gross or ordinary negligence; g) physical or mental impairments; h) drug or alcohol abuse

37. Every person is granted freedom from bodily contact by another person unless consent has been granted. Each diagnostic tests or intervention has different risks that must be conveyed to the client.
38. a) disclosure, b) comprehension, c) competence, and d) voluntariness
39. a) duty; b) breach of duty; c) causation; d) damages
40. a) don't discuss the case with anyone at your hospital except, in the US, nurses may discuss the case with the hospital's risk manager; b) don't discuss the case with the plaintiff; c) don't discuss the care with the plaintiff's lawyer; d) don't discuss the care with anyone testifying for the plaintiff; e) don't discuss the case with reporters; f) don't alter the patient's records; g) don't hide any information from your lawyer; g) don't go to the witness stand unprepared; h) don't be discourteous on the witness stand; i) don't volunteer any information
41. Programs which hospital and other health-care agencies have developed in an effort to reduce malpractice claims. These programs are designed to identify, analyze, and treat risks.
42. safety program, products safety program, quality assurance program.
43. a) respecting legal boundaries of practice; b) following institutional procedures and policies; c) "owning" personal strengths and weaknesses; d) evaluating proposed assignments; refusing to accept responsibilities for which one is not prepared; e) keeping current; f) respecting client rights and developing rapport with clients; g) keeping careful documentation; h) working within the institution to develop and support management policies

Unit II: The Client: Concepts for Holistic Care

Chapter 7: Human Needs

Key Terms Crossword Puzzle

Across	*Down*
1. sexuality	2. extended
3. cohabiting	3. community
6. esteem	4. belonging
7. blended	5. needs
8. basic human needs	9. actualization
11. nuclear	10. safety
12. physiologic	13. single
14. traditional	

Family Functions Table

14. Physical: provide safe, comfortable environment
15. Economic: financial aid for family members; monetary needs of society
16. Reproductive: birth of children
17. Affective/coping: emotional comfort and help members establish an identity and maintain that identity in the time of stress
18. Socialization: teaching; transmitting of beliefs, values, attitudes, and coping mechanisms; providing feedback and guidance in problem solving

Family Risk Factors

19. Biologic
20. Life-style
21. Social/Psychological
22. Social/Psychological
23. Social/Psychological
24. Life-style
25. Life-style
26. Biologic
27. Biologic
28. Social/Psychological
29. Environmental

Chapter 8: Culture and Ethnicity

Definitions

1. *humanism* concern and understanding of others which attests to the dignity and worth of all persons
2. *race* division of humans based on distinct physical characteristics
3. *ethnic group* minority groups that retain distinct customs, language, or social values as a result of a common heritage
4. *culture* sum total of human behavior or social characteristics peculiar to a specific group and passed from generation to generation, or from one to another within the group
5. *subculture* group of persons with different interests or goals than the primary group
6. *stereotyping* assigning characteristics to a group of people without considering specific individuality
7. *ethnocentrism* judgment of other people based on the standards and practices of one's own culture

Classification of Cultural Terms

Race : (8) white, (10) black, (16) yellow; Ethnic group: (9) Irish, (18) Mexican-Ameraican; Culture: (12) rural black, (14) Jewish, (15) urban poor; Subculture: (11) drug users, (13) steet people, (17) bag ladies

Poverty Defined:

19. Poverty is an economic lack; falling short of the money needed to purchase a minimum amount of goods and services
20. Poverty is relative; falling below the income level of the standards prevailing among individuals or in communities
21. Poverty is a relative lack of an individual's access to and control oven environmental resources.
22. Group: Reasons for Poverty
  a. female: Female heads of households are increasing and the woman often cannot earn enough money to meet the family's needs.
  b. elderly: Elderly people predominately depend on fixed incomes which do not keep pace with inflation
  c. minority groups: Minority groups have often been raised on poverty and find it difficult to escape the cycle; unemployment , feelings of despair, unstable families, and "escape" values such as drugs and alcohol are factors.

Race\Ethnic Group Match

23. B
24. A, F
25. A, D
26. G, H
27. A
28. F, D, A
29. A
30. A

Implementing

31. a) increase awareness of role of culture in own life; b) identify own biases and how they could affect care; c) learn about other cultures and their health care patterns; d) learn about people in own community with belief systems and practices different from your own; e) display accepting, non-judgmental attitudes with client's cultural beliefs

Chapter 9: Stress and Adaptation

Key Terms Scramblegram

1. adaptation
2. anxiety
3. burnout
4. coping mechanisms
5. crisis
6. intervention
7. defense mechanisms
8. developmental
9. "fight or flight"
10. Adaptation, GAS
11. homeostasis
12. inflammatory, reflex
13. local (LAS)
14. disorders
15. stress
16. stressor

Defense Mechanisms Match

17. C
18. I
19. F
20. H
21. E
22. B

Stress Short Answer

23. Exercise: helps maintain physical and emotional health through tension reduction, physiological benefits, and a sense of well-being
24. Rest and Sleep: allow the body to maintain homeostasis and restore energy levels; rest and energy act as insulation against stress
25. Nutrition: helps maintain the body's homeostatic mechanisms and increase resistance to stress

Crisis Intervention Steps

26. identify the problem
27. list alternatives
28. choose from among alternatives
29. implement a plan
30. evaluate the results

Physiologic Effects of Stress Match

31. B
32. A
33. D
34. C
35. D

Unit III: Promoting Wellness Across the Lifespan

Chapter 10: Developmental Concepts

Developmental Theories: Matching

1. H
2. G
3. A
4. I
5. J
6. C
7. E
8. F
9. D
10. B
11. I
12. G
13. F
14. C
15. H

16. J
17. B
18. D
19. E
20. A

Growth and Development Case Study

21. Tonio is showing some regression, probably due to the situational crises of the new baby in the family and possibly because of his father's absence from home. He also is in the phallic stage of Freud and could be expressing some of the Oedipus complex in his possessiveness of mom.
22. Initiative vs guilt -- Erikson
23. Sensorimotor stage -- Piage; primary circular reaction probably going to secondary circular reaction
24. Industry vs Inferiority -- Erikson
25. Concrete operational stage -- Piaget
26. Tell her what you are going to do and why she needs the shot. She will understand and accept this logically.
27. Tell her that children go through various stages of development of conscience and moral standards. Tonio is in the stage where rules are important. He learns acceptable standards of behavior through conformity to rules set by authority figures. When these are violated he feels guilty but he does not always understand the reason for the rule.
    Maria is in a different stage whereby she is able to understand the reason for the rules. She conforms more not so much out of fear of punishment but by the desire to identify with significant others and their ideals; she wants to be seen as a good girl.
28. Try again in a month or two. The timing will be better. The child probably pushed at the food because of the extrusion reflex. She should be more amenable to spoon feeding after it has disappeared.
29. Generativity vs Stagnation -- Erikson
30. Postconventional -- Kohlberg
31. Conflicts will most likely arise especially when she is trying to meet the needs of so many at such different developmental levels as well as her own. She may need help setting priorities.
32. The family unit can have both positive and negative influences on each individual member's development. Good family relationships and healthy environments are important to help facilitate this.

Chapter 11: Conception to Midlife

Pre-Embryonic Development

1. A
2. C
3. B
4. B
5. C
6. B
7. A
8. B
9. B

Adult Development

10. A
11. B
12. D
13. F
14. C
15. E

Childhood Development: Completion

16. a. 3 mo.; b. 4 mo; c. 5 mo.; d. 8 mo.; e. 6 mo
17. 1 min. and 5 min.
18. a. heart rate; b. respiratory rate; c. muscle tone; d. reflex irritability; e. color
19. It was designed to identify through neurologic and behavioral assessment subtle differences in the way infants respond to their surroundings. Involves complex performance of activities of the infant and measurable activities such as alertness, muscle tone, sleep-wake patterns, reflexes, etc.
20. birth to 28 days
21. a. congenital malformations
    b. respiratory distress syndrome
    c. incompatible blood group
    d. birth trauma
22. A screening tool for the infant/child to pick up atypical developmental patterns that may need more precise assessment and follow-up.
23. a. gross motor development; b. fine motor development; c. language development; d. personal/social interaction
24. Bonding - initial fusing ie. mother-child response
    Attachment - long term maintenance of relationship
25. Traits visible in infancy remain consistent into adulthood. Three outstanding temperaments: Easy (positive), Difficult (negative), and Slow to warm (variable range).
    Easy - Easiest to care for, rhythmic behavior, smiles, sociable, agreeable to work with.
    Slow to warm - Takes more work to encourage responses, may be more passive, not as overtly responsive.
    Difficult - Intense reactions, more difficult to deal with ie. restless sleeper, sensitive to noise, dif-

ficulty with self control as a toddler, poor eater, possible colicky baby.

26. a) Separation anxiety; b) Fear of pain or bodily mutilation
27. Interest in the opposite sex limited. Identification with one's own sex dominant. Psychosocial energies channeled in other directions. School-age 6-12 years, middle childhood.
28. It is a relatively quiet period. Growth is slow and steady. There are no major upheavals or crises present.
29. preconventional; conventional
30. a) Good-boy, Good-girl orientation in that they like to please others: b) Law and order orientation (respect for the law)
31. A relationship of reciprocal fairness.
32. a) Sex-object preference; b) Sex-role behavior
33. a.- f. Your answer should include six of the following: Achieve new and more mature relationships; Achieve masculine/feminine social role; Accept one's physique; Acquire a set of values and an ethical system; Desire and achieve socially responsible behavior; Achieve emotional independence; Prepare for a long term heterosexual relationship; Prepare for a career
34. a) Accidents; b) Homicide; c) Suicide
35. Intimacy vs. Isolation
36. Characteristics of Intimacy vs Isolation include: a) Select life partner; b) Choose an occupation/career; c) Establish intimate relationships; d) Establish independence from parents; e) Establish a social network; f) Form a personal philosophical and ethical structure
37. Generativity vs. Stagnation
38. a) Establish and guide the next generation; b) Accept middle age changes; c) Adjust to needs of aging parents; d) Being comfortable with spouse; e) Reevaluate goals and accomplishments
39. a) Choosing a vocation; b) Defining relationship choices
40. Demands increase from needs of aging parents/other family members while children increasing in independence may still require assistance or have demands on parents. Balancing these requirements and requests with meeting their own needs and desires may be tricky.
41. a) Motor vehicular accidents; b) Occupational accidents; c) Suicide; d) Chronic disease: cancer in women and heart attacks in men
42. a) Self; b) The cultural aspects of one's life; c) The particular set of roles in which one participates; It has to completely reorganize
43. Transformation

Clinical Situations

44. B
45. A
46. C
47. A
48. C
49. B
50. A
51. A
52. B
53. B
54. C
55. No, probably not. Viability before the 6th month is not likely.
56. Breasts enlarge; increased oxygen consumption; abdominal breathing changes to thoracic breathing; Increased blood volume; Decreased gastric emptying time and decreased intestinal motility; Increased size of uterus causing pressure on the kidneys, ureters, and bladder; Skin pigmentations; Accentuated lumbosacral spinal curve, postural changes as uterus grows; Weight gain of 25-30 pounds; Increased water retention; Increased carbohydrate and iron needs
57. Learn about physical and psychological changes of pregnancy; Accept his supportive role in meeting the needs of his wife; understand sexual alterations and activity during pregnancy; Explore feelings about the developing infant; Learn about the birthing process; Accept own feelings about the actual birth;
58.

Hazards/NursesRole:

Accidents: Provide information on safety in the work place and in activities of daily living,

Relationships - 1) Sex experimentation, 2) Childbirth, 3) Diseases, etc.: Provide information on birth control, pregnancy, STD's etc. Reproductive health

Drug and substance abuse: Teach regarding dangers of substance abuse and available programs

Diet and Exercise - 1) Obesity; 2) Nutritional problems; 3) Over and under exercise problems: Teach regarding stress management, rest, good nutrition and safe exercise activities, etc.

59. D
60. A
61. Andropause
62. Maintain desired weight; Proper nutrition; Moderate exercise; Regular blood pressure checks; Stop smoking; Watch alcohol consumption; Annual physical and dental exams; regular eye exams; Routine exams for cancer, breast, mammogram, Pap tests, prostate and testes, colon; Rest and relax!

Chapter 12: The Older Adult
Case Study Short Answer
1. She should speak clearly and slowly, look directly at the client, repeat instructions, listen carefully to him, insure adequate lighting to see one another communicating. Assess for potential effectiveness of hearing aid.
2. Cognition does not change appreciably with aging. However, speed of processing and responding may decrease. Mild short-term memory loss may occur but can be remedied by note-taking and calendars.
3. Seems to have adjusted to declining physical strength and health and to retirement and loss of his spouse to some degree. Has not however adjusted to adopting new social roles and affiliations. He may also need assistance with housekeeping and meals.
4. In Ego integrity vs Despair. Listening helps an older person review his life and achieve ego integrity.
5. Association of Retired Persons; Senior Citizens Housing; Area Agency on Aging; Senior Homemaker Services; Parks and Recreation Senior Adult Programs; Senior Nutrition Sites

Chapter 13:Loss, Grief, and Death
Key Terms Match
1. D
2. B
3. H
4. A
5. G
6. J
7. E
8. C
9. F
10. I

True and False
11. False
12. True
13. False
14. True
15. False
16. False

Unit IV: Nursing Process

Chapter 14: Introduction to Nursing Process
Nursing Process Match
1. B, C
2. A, D, E
3. A, B
4. A
5. D
6. A, B
7. E
8. C
9. B
10. E
11. D
12. B

Chapter 15: Assessing
Completion
1. introduction
2. nursing history
3. systematic
4. developmental
5. comprehensive
6. medical
7. validate
8. assessment
9. subjective
10. termination
11. documentation
12. objective
13. observation

Chapter 16: Diagnosing
Nursing Diagnoses: Match
1. B
2. Correct
3. A
4. C
5. A
6. Correct
7. D
8. Correct
9. D
10. Correct
11. E
12. G
13. F
14. F
15. Correct

16. E
17. Correct
18. E, G
19. H
20. E
21. Correct
22. F
23. E
24. F, G
25. F

Chapter 17: Planning

Client Goals Categorized

1. cognitive
2. affective
3. psychomotor
4. psychomotor
5. cognitive

Writing Goal Statements

6 A C B D.
7. A B C.
8. C A C B C.
9. C A B C D.

Guidelines for Selecting Nursing Actions

10-12. The nursing orders selected must be:

a. Tailored to the client
b. Consistent with standards of care
c. Realistic in terms of abilities, time, and resources
d. Compatible with client's values, beliefs, and psychosocial background
e. Valued by client and nurse
f. Compatible with other planned therapies

Writing Nursing Orders: Sentence Completion

Comprehensive nursing orders include:

13. nursing observations
14. nursing actions/activities/measures
15. teaching, counseling
16. on-going

Nursing Kardex

Nursing care related to:

17. nursing diagnoses
18. the medical plan of care
19. basic human needs

Nursing Actions Related to Diagnosis

Sleep pattern disturbance r/t pain and anxiety....

20. Sleep pattern disturbance
21. Sleep pattern disturbance
22. r/t pain and anxiety
23. Sleep pattern disturbance
24. r/t pain and anxiety

Chapter 18: Implementing/Documenting-Documentation

1. Ct has been OOB 2X this shift. C/O mild pain in abd. on amb., but no pallor or SOB. O2 dc'd at 9:00 a.m. Homan's sign neg. BP, P and R WNL. Abd. soft, not distended; bowel sounds auscultated X 4 quadrants. No BM today. Reminded ct to void in receptacle for measurement of I & O.
2. Communication Methods and Disadvantages

Face-to-face meeting: ordinarily there is no permanent record for later use; both the sending and receiving persons must be available at the same time, in the same place

Telephone conversation: ordinarily there is no permanent record for later use; no nonverbal message can be given; only the tone of voice and voice inflections can be communicated

Written message: message usually cannot be validated with the sender; no nonverbal messages can be given

Audiotaped message: message usually cannot be validated with sender; no nonverbal message can be given; only the tone of voice and inflection can be communicated

3. Guidelines for Care

A. Before implementing any nursing action, reassess the client to determine if the action is still needed. The client situation may have changed since initial assessment.

B. Approach the client competently. Know how to perform the nursing action, why the action is being performed, and potential adverse responses. Have all equipment and supplies ready. The nurse is accountable for safe, competent care. Competence increases client security and quality of care.

C. Approach the client caringly. Compassion and caring increase trust and client security.

Chapter 19: Evaluating

Evaluation Standards and Criteria

1. C
2. C
3. S
4. S
5. C

Factors Impacting on Quality of Nursing Care

6. Inadequate staffing: Develop/use a patient classification system that identifies kind and number of nursing services needed. Record staffing patterns and relate to nursing care and patient outcomes. Document that adequate staffing

makes a difference.Present to nursing administration with request for additional staff.

7. Boredom, loss of interest in nursing: Identify personal objectives related to work. Explore avenues for professional growth. Initiate changes to stimulate improved care. Participate in committees, programs, institutional projects. Explore other career development options/positions.
8. Inadequate supplies: Identify and clearly document problems with obtaining supplies. Enlist support of other units. Talk with nursing administration suggesting potential corrective strategies.

Data Correlated to Type of Evaluation

9. Outcome
10. Process
11. Process
12. Structure
13. Structure
14. Outcome

Unit V: Roles Basic to Nursing Practice

Chapter 20: Communicator

Communication: True False

1. True
2. True
3. False
4. False
5. True
6. True
7. False

Communication and the Nursing Process

8. a) data collection: read written word--chart; verbal history; written communication in Kardex and chart; verbal & nonverbal interaction
   b) diagnosis: communication to other nurses & to client; written communication of diagnosis in Kardex and chart
   c) planning: verbal communication with client and other nurses; written communication of plan in Kardex and chart
   d) implementation: verbal & non verbal communication in care, e.g., teaching, counseling,supporting, coordinating; written communication in chart
   e) evaluation: verbal & nonverbal communication with nurses & clients; written communication in chart
9. a) It is dynamic; b) It is purposeful & time-limited; c) Person providing assistance assumes dominant role and responsibility
10. Discuss/acknowledge goal achievement; set the stage for transition to other staff/home; encourage expression of feelings related to termination

Communication Match

11. G
12. F
13. C
14. D
15. E

Communication Crossword Puzzle

Across	*Down*
1. touch	1. posture
2. words	2. body language
3. eye contact	3. silence
4. gestures	4. facial
5. dress	5. sounds
	6. tactile

Chapter 21: Teacher/Counselor

Teaching Role of the Nurse: Short Answer

1. Trends in health care have made the role of teacher more important: shorter hospital stays mean clients need more extensive home-care information and more thorough in-patient teaching prior to discharge. A shorter time period means quality must be improved. Also, shortened hospital stays increase the need for community health nurses with teaching and counseling skills in assisting clients adjust to acute care situations at home.
2. teaching: a planned method or series of methods used to help someone learn
3. learning: the process by which a person acquires or increases knowledge or changes behavior in a measurable way
4. situational crisis: occurs when a client faces an event or situation that causes a disruption in life
5. developmental crisis: occurs when a person is going through a life passage or developmental stage

Teaching/Learning True and False

6. False
7. True
8. False
9. True

Teaching Assessment

10. Developmental level --
    Affects what & how people learn. Affects teaching strategies.
11. Level of Education --

Important to teaching approaches & kind of content presented.

12. Emotional health --
 Affects client's ability to receive and process information.
13. Self-image --
 Affects client's ability and desire to learn
14. Culture --
 Affects how the teaching/learning process is perceived. May affect content presented and teaching approaches.

Evaluation of Teaching

15. All of the following can be used to determine if teaching-learning goals have been achieved: direct questioning; observation of patient behavior; return demonstration; home health care nurse feedback

Teaching Strategies: Matching

16. E
17. C
18. D
19. A
20. B

Counseling Completion

21. situational
22. developmental
23. short-term
24. long-term
25. motivational

Learning Domains

26. Cognitive Domain: categorizes, defines, explains, lists, states
27. Affective Domain: chooses, defends,helps, justifies, shares
28. Psychomotor Domain: arranges, assembles, constructs, shows
29. a) explains; b) shows; c) chooses

Chapter 22: Leader/Research/Advocate

1-5. You might have listed such things as enthusiastic, self-directed, good role model, self-comfort and confidence, positive self-image, intelligent, warm, flexible, effective communication skills, hard-working, honest.

6. C
7. B
8. A
9. A

Crossword Puzzle

Across	*Down*
2. extraneous	1. traditional
4. authoritative	3. data
7. scientific	5. variables
8. dependent	6. research
9. control	7. study

Advocate Role: Short Answer

10. a. Talk with husband and wife about the colostomy and resources in the community where they can receive help.
 b. Make referrals to a colostomy support group.
 c. Make a referral for some post-discharge home visits.

Advocacy: True/False

11. True
12. False
13. False
14. True
15. False
16. False
17. True

Unit VI:Actions Basic to Nursing Practice

Chapter 23: Vital Signs

1. E
2. J
3. C
4. K
5. D
6. F
7. A
8. B
9. I
10. G

Vital Sign: Paragraph Definitions

11. *sphygmomanometer:* equipment used for obtaining an indirect measure of blood pressure; consists of an inflatable cuff and a manometer, which is a mercury-filled cylinder calibrated in millimeters
12. *vital signs*: cardinal signs which provide an indication of the physiologic functioning of the body; reflected in temperature, pulse, respirations and blood pressure.
13. *pyrexic*: having a body temperature elevated above normal
14. *pulse rate*: the sensation caused in an artery each time the left ventricle of the heart contracts to eject blood into the aorta, thereby causing an increase in pressure and an expansion of the arterial walls
15. *tachypneic*: having a respiratory rate faster than normal
16. *systolic pressure*: the highest pressure exerted on the arterial walls caused by the left ventricle of

the heart contracting and pushing blood through the aortic valve

17. *diastolic pressure*: the lowest pressure exerted on the arterial walls following the contraction of the heart

Vital Sign:Completion

18. hypothalamus
19. circadian rhythm
20. hyperpyrexia
21. conduction
22. lubricated
23. orthostatic hypotension
24. auscultation
25. radial artery
26. pulse pressure
27. arm

Chapter 24: Nursing Assessment

Key Terms Match

1. I
2. M
3. L
4. A
5. B
6. F
7. D
8. E
9. J
10. K
11. C
12. H
13. G
14. N

Positioning for Physical Examination

15-20. Compare your drawings with those in your text, Fundamentals of Nursing, page 436, Figure 24-3 (Taylor, 1988)

Cranial Nerve Assessment

21. I *Olfactory* - sensory; sense of smell
22. II *Optic* - sensory: sense of vision
23. III *Oculomotor* - motor: pupil constriction, raise eyelids
24. IV *Trochlear* - motor: downward inward eye movement
25. V *Trigeminal* - motor: jaw movements--chewing and mastication; sensory: sensation on the face and neck
26. VI *Abducens* - motor: lateral movement of the eyes
27. VII *Facial* - motor: muscles of the face; sensory: sense of taste on the anterior two thirds of the tongue
28. VIII *Acoustic* - sensory: sense of hearing
29. IX *Glossopharyngeal* - motor: pharyngeal movement and swallowing; sensory: sense of taste on the posterior one third of the tongue
30. X *Vagus* - motor: swallowing and speaking
31. XI *Spinal accessory* - motor; movement of shoulder muscles
32. XII *Hypoglossal* - motor: movement of the tongue and strength of the tongue

Chapter 25: Safety and Asepsis

Key Terms Match

1. E
2. B
3. A
4. D
5. G
6. E
7. F
8. H
9. I
10. L
11. K
12. J

Accident Proofing

13. kitchen: You might suggest checking the condition of the pilot light and securing the stove knobs out of the reach of children; chairs proper height and repair; storage areas easily reached; condition of floors, eg.; adequacy of lighting; mats/rugs nonskid; knives and sharp instruments out of reach of children; cleaning chemicals out of reach of children.
14. living room: You might suggest stairways being secured from children falling; rooms uncluttered to permit easy mobility; electrical outlets secured so that children cannot put sharp instruments in them.
15. bedroom: You might suggest checking the accessibility of light switches; adequacy of lighting; bed and chairs of adequate height.
16. bathroom: You might suggest placing mat or skidproof strips in tub/shower; illuminated medication cabinet secured from access by children.
17. Porch and yard: You might suggest checking to see that sidewalks and steps are in good repair with handrails securely fastened; adequate lighting; holes and wells filled in.

Infectious Disease Table Completion

18-27. Compare your answers with those in Table 25-8 of your Fundamentals of Nursing text (Taylor, 1988, 522)

Chapter 26: Admitting, Discharge and Home Visits

Client Admission

1. Position the bed in its highest position.
2. Clear the furniture and bedside table to allow room for the stretcher to enter.
3. Fold back the bedspread, blanket, and top sheet.
4. Assemble equipment and supplies: admission pack, gown, blood pressure equipment.
5. Obtain an IV standard

Patient Teaching

6. Medication - The client will know: drug name; what dosage to take and when; purpose of drug; effect(s) the drug should have; symptoms of possible adverse effects, and which ones to report.
7. Environment - The client will be assured of: adequate instruction in necessary homemaking skills; investigation and correction of any physical hazards in the home environment; adequate emotional support; investigation of sources of economic support; investigation of transportation means to appointments and/or clients.
8. Treatment - The client and family will: know the purpose of any treatment to be continued at home; be able to demonstrate correct performance of the treatment.
9. Health Teaching - The client will: describe how his or her disease or condition affects body function; describe the means necessary to maintain present level of health, or achieve a higher level of health.
10. Outpatient Referral - The client will: know when and where to keep clinical appointments; know where and whom to call for medical help; take home written discharge instuctions.
11. Diet - The client will be able to: describe the purpose of his or her prescribed diet; plan several typical menus using the prescribed diet.

Home Visit Assessment

12. What is the financial status of this family? Are finances adequate for needs (food, rent, utilities)? How much more is needed for added medication and supply costs? Do they have insurance: What carrier do they have and how much is reimbursed? Is the family in need of assistance? Are they eligible for food stamps, rent and energy rebates, medication subsidy?

Discharge Planning

13. must be coordinated
14. must be interdisciplinary
15. must be initiated as early as possible
16. must be carefully planned
17. must involve client, family or significant others

UNIT VII: Promoting Healthy Physiologic Responses

Chapter 27 Hygiene

Developmental Factors Affecting Skin Condition

1. Infant: Skin and mucous membranes easily injured and subject to infection.
2. Child: Skin increasingly resistant; requires special care because of toilet and play habits.
3. Adolescent: Skin has enlarged sebaceous glands and increased secretions which predispose to acne.
4. Older Individual: Skin becomes thinner and less elastic. Subcutaneous fat decreases predisposing to injury. Skin becomes dry due to decreased oil secretion.
5. Reduces fatigue; maintains warmth; promotes clean, fresh feeling; and decreases dry, itchy skin.
6. Place large towel in bag and soak with warm cleaning agent; wring out well and unroll towel on client while removing linens; fold extra towel under client's chin for later use; beginning with feet use massaging motion to clean body; fold towel upward as bath proceeds; cleanse facial area with extra towel under chin; fold towel into quarters with soiled side in and use folded towel to wash back and buttocks; remove towel and rub back; client need not be dried.
7. To prevent phlebitis and thrombi formation by forcing blood in superficial veins to deeper veins and preventing stagnation and pooling of blood in leg veins.
8. Explain rationale for use; wash hands; be sure stockings fit by measuring; assist client to supine position; provide privacy; expose legs one at a time and powder or lotion to make application easier; bunch stockings to heel; ease over client's toes, foot, and heel; grasp and pull up smoothly and straight.
9. a) *Dry skin*: Causes may include dry climate; soap or alcohol residue; inadequate fluid intake. Should bathe less when dry; rinse skin and clothes well ; increase fluids; use an emollient.

   b) *Acne:* Causes may include hormones; oil-based cosmetics or lotions; certain foods such as cola and chocolate. Should wash skin and hair with soap and hot water; avoid oily products; avoid aggravating foods.

   c) *Skin rashes:* Causes may include contact with an allergen or systemic responses to medications, foods, diseases. Should wash with mild cleansing agent and rinse well; use antiseptic or cream to reduce inflammation and itchying; avoid allergens.

10. a) File toenails as opposed to cutting; do not cut or use commercial remover for corns or calluses; avoid stockings or positions which cut off blood flow; keep feet warm and dry; do not go bare foot; break in new shoes very gradually.
b) Bathe feet thoroughly in soap and water; rinse well; soak if toenails are thick and brittle; trim or file nails straight across; apply powder or lanolin cream.

Key Terms: Match

11. E
12. D
13. H
14. A
15. C
16. F
17. G
18. B
19. I
20. N
21. M
22. J
23. K
24. L

Chapter 28: Activity

Body Position: Match

1. E
2. C
3. J
4. G
5. I
6. F
7. B
8. H
9. D
10. A
11. M
12. K
13. X
14. O
15. W
16. U
17. L
18. S
19. N
20. V
21. T
22. P
23. R
24. Q

Crossword Puzzle

Across	*Down*
3. active	1. osteoporosis
5. paraplegia	2. Fowler's
6. contractures	3. atrophy
8. synovial	4. sims
12. tonus	7. spastic
14. isotonic	9. orthopedics
15. flaccid	10. ankylosis
16. ADL	11. passive
17. isometric	13. semi Fowler's
19. stretching	15. aerobic
21. isokinetic	18. ROM
22. prone	20. dangle

Short Answer

25. a) developmental considerations; b) physical health; c) mental health; d) life-style variables; e) attitude and values; f) fatigue/stress; g) external factors, eg. weather, financial resources, air pollution, etc.
26. a) develop a habit of erect posture; b) use the longest and strongest muscles of the arms and legs to provide power for strenuous activities; c) use internal girdle and long midriff to stabilize the pelvis; d) work as close as possible to an object that is to be lifted or moved; e) use the weight of the body as a force for pulling or pushing; f) place the feet apart to provide a wider base of support when increased stability of the body is necessary; g) flex the knees, use the internal girdle, and come down close to an object that is to be lifted.
27. a) consistently utilize sound principles of body mechanics; b) incorporate regular periods of exercise into life-style; c) demonstrate a preference for an active vs. sedentary life-style; d) appear physically fit to clients and colleagues.
28. General ease of movement and gait; alignment, joint structure, and function; muscle mass, tone, and strength; and endurance.
29. Teach client what is being undertaken and why; avoid over-exhaustion; start gradually and work slowly; move each joint until there is resistance but not pain; support joints and muscles to prevent strain; return joint to a neutral position; keep friction at a minimum; use ROM 2-3 times a day regularly.
30. Know client's capabilities and place devices before trying to move; plan carefully what will be done and enlist help if needed; explain to client what you plan and how he can assist; give pain med in advance of moving if needed; remove obstacles, elevate bed as

necessary; lock any wheels being used; use good body mechanics; support client in good alignment; avoid friction; move smoothly.

31. They are isometric exercises which help reduce weakness and make walking easier for bedridden clients. The client should prepare for ambulation by contracting the muscles on the front of the thighs by pushing the backs of the knees into the bed and pulling feet upward.
32. Client sits at side of bed without feeling faint, stands a moment, takes deep breaths, looks ahead, walks a short distance with assistance or nurse at side
33. Measure by having client lie flat in bed on back wearing walking shoes; measure from anterior fold of axilla straight down to heel and add 5 cm; have client stand to adjust handgrips when crutches obtained; teach client that support of body weight should be mostly on hands and arms. Prepare client with arm and shoulder strengthening exercises.
34. a) *Four-point gait*: weight bearing permitted on both feet; b) *Two-point gait*: weight-bearing permtted on both feet with more speed than four-point gait; c) *Three-point gait:* weight-bearing is permitted on only one foot with other foot not supporting but balancing; d) *Swing-through gait:* weight-bearing is permitted on only one foot with no assist of other foot (if present) or can be used by paraplegic with weight on both feet.
35. Explore client's fitness goals, interests, skills capacity; assist in obtaining medical clearance; explore feasible exercises with client regarding time, equipment, risk, etc.; develop exercise program; identify potential threats and supports; evaluate.
36. Support pillows are needed for correct positioning. Areas of the body needing attention are the arm and leg on the side opposite the one on which the person is lying. Place pillows under head and neck, top arm, top leg from groin to foot. Provide hand-wrist splint if needed. Align shoulders with hips.
37. a) Impaired physical mobility related to pain b) Nutritional alterations: more than body requirements related to imbalance between calories ingested and "burned off" c) Potential for further injury related to muscle wasting and past history.

Chapter 29: Rest and Sleep

Key Terms Match

1. H
2. O
3. C
4. J
5. U
6. G
7. D
8. N
9. P
10. A
11. F
12. T
13. M
14. R
15. B
16. K
17. R
18. P
19. I
20. E
21. L

Case Study

22. a) Be sure you have considered his developmental stage, reduction in physical activity, psychologic stress, dietary patterns, obesity, hypertension, and sexual assessment (refer to text, p. 694, 698, 702).
    b) Sleep pattern disturbance, excessive daytime sleepiness related to disturbed nocturnal sleep secondary to sleep apnea (see text, p. 705-706).
    c) The client will demonstrate decreased signs of sleep deprivation by 3/8 (refer to text, p. 707).
    d) Develop your goals with Geneva's need to understand the underlying causes of sleep apnea.
    e) Obesity is a risk factor in sleep apnea. Airway obstruction is more likely to occur in the supine position.
    f) (Refer to text, p. 707).
    g) (Refer to text, p. 710 for ideas).
    h) Base your answer upon the specific article you have found.
    i) Steve's signs and symptoms of sleep deprivation will have diminished or abated.
23. a) noise reduced, lighting off or subdued; temperature moderate (refer to text p. 698-699).
    b) (Refer to text, p. 698 for ideas).
    c) Consider those activities which create noise or motion in your answer.
    d) Have you considered the stages of sleep in your answer?
    e) Individualize, based upon clients' assessed normal sleep-wake patterns.
    f) Promote relaxation/restful environment, promote bedtime rituals, provide bedtime snack.
    g) Nutritional aspects are essential to be considered, especially related to protein intake.

Chapter 30: Comfort

Match

1. C
2. J
3. A, I
4. B, C
5. F
6. G
7. D
8. A, H
9. A, I
10. I
11. B

Pain Syndromes

12. J
13. D
14. A
15. E
16. B
17. E
18. C
19. H
20. G

Analgesia

21. Morphine: CNS mech. blocks pain stimulus to brain; n/v, sedation, resp. depression; yes
22. Demerol: CNS mech. blocks pain stimulus to brain; n/v, sedation, resp. depression; yes
23. Aspirin: blocks prostaglandin synthesis; n/v, gastric distress, inhibits coagulation; no

Patient Goal Statements

24. Family will demonstrate ability to discuss pain experience and offer emotional support to client.
25. Client will demonstrate ability to perform ADL's while using pain control methods as taught.
26. Client will describe a gradual reduction in pain using a scale of 0-10
27. Client will demonstrate willingness to take prescribed analgesic by asking for medication without prompting from staff
28. Client will demonstrate means of controlling pain while continuing to cough and deep breathe.

Pain Responses

29. C
30. B
31. B
32. C
33. A
34. A
35. B
36. C
37. C
38. A
39. B
40. B
41. C
42. A
43. B
44. C

Key Term Definitions

45. Analgesia - a medication which reduces pain by either blocking pain stimulus at level of CNS or by inhibiting prostaglandin synthesis
    b. Diffuse Pain - pain that covers a large area
    c. Pain Tolerance - the ability to withstand or cope with pain
    d. Pain Threshold - the point at which a person recognizes a stimulus as painful
    e. Psychogenic Pain - pain having a mental rather than physical origin

Crossword

Across	*Down*
1. sharp	1. severe
2. excruciating	2. dull
3. contralateral	3. referred
4. acupuncture	4. acupuncture
5. imagery	5. placebo
6. somatic	6. acute
7. help	7. hypnosis
8. endorphins	8. comfort
9. chronic	9. ease
10. relax	10. visceral
11. tens	11. mild
	12. phantom
	13. calm
	14. pain

Chapter 31: Nutrition

Nutrition Terms

1. D
2. F
3. I
4. G
5. J
6. A
7. C
8. E
9. B
10. H

Nutrition Completion

11. lipids; carbohydrates; proteins
12. thiamine
13. vitamin A
14. potassium
15. sodium

Nutrition Crossword Puzzle

Across	*Down*
2. bulimia	2. bran

35. anorexia
76. amino acid
87. RDA
106. salem
112. calorie
143. CHO
196. ECF
203. ICF
213. ATP
233. set point

6. mineral
27. water
49.TPN
61.fat soluble
68. disaccharide
108. lipid
110. MAC
118. EGG
198. FAT

Nutrition Case Study
16. 108-121 lb.
17. Methods:
    a. (115 x 10 = 1150) + (115 x 5 = 575) = 1725 calories
    b. 115 x 15 = 1725 calories
    c. 115 x 18 = 2070 calories
18. 1600-2400 calories/day

The Nurse as a Critical Thinker
19. Put tube in ice water for 5-10 minutes before inserting it.
10. Measure NG tube from tip of nose to earlobe and from his earlobe to his xiphoid process - marking with tape.
21. Inject 10-20 cc of air into NG tube & auscultate over epigastric area with a stethoscope.
22. Aspirate stomach contents before the beginning of each feeding.
23. Elevate the patient's bed at least 30 degrees.
24. Introduce 30-60 cc of water after all the feeding is given.
25. Discontinue the suction on the machine.
26. Clamp tube with fingers while removing tube.

Nutritional Substances
27. iron, iodine, zinc
28. calcium, phosphorus, magnesium
29. egg yolk, animal fats
30. meat, milk, beans, cheese
31. bread, rice, potatoes
32. iodized salt, seafood
33. bran, whole grain bread, raw fruits & vegetables
34. glucose, fructose, galactose
35. sunflower, soybean, corn oils
36. legumes, bananas, potatoes, tomatoes

Chapter 32: Bowel Elimination

Elimination: Match
1. F
2. E
3. G
4. H
5. B
6. K
7. A
8. I
9. D
10. C

Large Intestine: Completion
11. ileocecal valve
12. anus
13. 3 inches
14. 1 inch
15. 800 cc
16. 1000 cc
17. sigmoid
18. rectum
19. anal canal
20. sphincter
21. autonomic
22. defecation

Bowel Elimination Case Study
23. Diagnosis: alteration in bowel elimination: constipation RT stress, aging, lack of proper foods and adequate fluids.
24. Goals: (a) Mr. Cranby will have soft, formed bowels movements every 1-2 days. (b) Mr. Cranby will verbalize the importance of fiber and fluid in his diet and its relationship to adequate bowel movements.
25. Nursing Interventions:
    a. at least 8 glasses of water daily
    b. fiber in diet
    c. stool softener prn
    d. regular daily exercise
    e. laxative as needed
    f. relaxation exercises daily
    g. privacy during bowel movements

Bowel Elimination Crossword Puzzle

Across
15. fiber
25. guiac
54. odor
58. ileus
64. distention
97. peristalsis
130. sims
138. sympathetic
153. mom
194. codeine
223. rectum
237. sitz

Down
9. valsalva
16. iron
21. polyp
33. ugi

56. ostomy
98. enema
138. stool
148. chyme
153. motor
180. anus
188. water

Bowel Elimination Problem Identification

26. paralytic ileus
27. fecal impaction
28. diarrhea
29. flatulence
30. incontinence

Enema Classification

31. RF
32. R
33. C
34. C
35. R
36. C

GI Jeopardy

37. What is a rectal foley catheter?
38. What are hemorrhoids?
39. What is the proper routine for collection of a stool specimen?
40. What are pinworms?
41. What is an esophagogastroduodenoscopy?
42. What foods should this client with an ostomy stay away from?
43. What is mineral oil?
44. What is an oil retention enema?
45. What is a rectal suppository?
46. What is a stoma?
47. What is an irrigation?

Chapter 33: Urinary Elimination

Urinary Elimination Diagnostic Procedures: Match

1. B
2. C
3. A
4. A
5. A,C
6. B,C
7. A

Urinary Medication: Completion

8. Prevent the reabsorption of water and certain electrolytes in the renal tubules
9. Stimulate contraction of the detrusor muscle & produce urination
10. Diminish the effectiveness of the neural reflex which interferes with the ability to urinate
11. same as analgesics

Urine Specimen Collection: Completion

12. sterile
13. appearance
14. clean-catch; catheterizing; indwelling catheter
15. all; 24-hour
16. voids; mid-stream; discarded
17. sterile
18. glucose; ketones
19. collected; bladder
20. glucose; protein; bilirubin; blood
21. drainage bag; analysis

Urinary Elimination Crossword Puzzle

Across:

1. frequency
2. polyuria
3. urge
4. urgency
5. stoma
6. catheter
7. anuria
8. dysuria
9. ileal conduit
10. incontinence

Down:

1. enuresis
2. cystoscopy
3. reflex
4. nocturia
5. hesitancy
6. irrigation
7. suppression
8. pyuria

Urinary Terms: Word Scramble and Definition

22. Glycosuria: presence of sugar in the urine
23. Orthostatic albuminuria: presence of albumin in urine that is voided after standing, walking, or running
24. Hematuria: blood in the urine
25. Retention: inability to void although urine is produced by the kidneys
26. Proteinuria: albumin in the urine
27. Oliguria: scanty or greatly diminished amount of urine voided in a given time
28. Pneumaturia: passage of urine containing gas
29. Dysuria: painful urination

Incontinence: Match

30. C
31. E
32. C
33. A
34. D
35. B
36. B
37. A
38. E
39. C

Urinary Elimination Definition of Terms

40. hydrometer: an instrument which measures the density of a liquid by the depth to which a graduated scale sinks into the liquid
41. micturition: the voiding of urine
42. residual urine: urine left in the bladder after urination
43. suprapubic catheter: a tube inserted into a surgical opening of the bladder above the symphysis pubis
44. urinometer: device for determining urine's specific gravity
45. voiding: evacuation of the bladder
46. Foley catheter: a tube used for bladder drainage and irrigation, which maintains its position in the bladder by the inflation of a balloon with sterile water

Characteristics of Urine

47. color: from straw colored to amber depending on concentration
48. odor: aromatic, develops odor of ammonia as it stands
49. turbidity: clear or translucent
50. pH: normal range is from 4.6 to 8
51. specific gravity: range of 1.10 to 1.025
52. constituents: primarily urea, uric acid, creatinine, ammonia, sodium, and chloride, primarily

Chapter 34: Oxygenation

Key Terms Match

1. C
2. G
3. H
4. A
5. J
6. I
7. B
8. E
9. D
10. F

Nursing Examination of the Respiratory System: Completion

11. anterior-posterior; transverse; symmetrical
12. trachea; 5 to 8 cm
13. resonance; hyperresonance; dullness
14. with his mouth open; nasal; adventitious

Oxygen Treatment

15. nasal cannula
16. nasal catheter
17. partial rebreathing mask
18. nonrebreathing mask
19. Venturi mask
20. oxygen tent

Pulmonary Function Tests

21. *Tidal Volume:* 500 ml inspired and expired during a normal respiration
22. *IRV:* this air is inspired beyond a normal breath - 3500-4300 ml
23. *ERV:* 1200-1500 ml is this amount that can be expired after a normal expiration
24. *VC:* after a maximal inspiration, this is the maximal amount of air a person can expire - 4000-4800 ml
25. *FVC:* after a fast maximal force expiration, this is the maximal amount of inspired air - 4800 ml
26. *FRC:* this is the sum of the ERV and RV. It can range from 2400-3000 ml
27. *RV:* this is the air that's still in the lungs after a maximal expiration
28. *TLC:* the sum of the tidal volume and the residual volume about 5500 ml

Respiratory Crossword Puzzle

Across

20. perfusion
81. rhonchi
93. IPPB
115. IRV
150. oxygenation
179. xray
201. dyspnea
225. Staph
234. rale

Down

6. bronchoscopy
11. bodycell
25. smoking
35. hypoxia
77. vibration
81. RV
181. ACTH
203. SOAP
207. ABGS

Respiratory Jeopardy.

The Question is.....

29. Where is the pleural space?
30. What is diffusion of gases?
31. What is ventilation?
34. What are alveoli?
35. What is the respiratory nursing history?
36. What is a pleural friction rub?
37. What is a problem statement?
38. What are expectorants?
39. What is an endotracheal tube?
40. What are the ABC's of basic life support?
41. What is two-rescuer CPR?
42. What is a skin test?

Chapter 35: Fluid, Electrolyte, and Acid-Base Balance

1- 5. Functions of Water in the Body (any 5 of the items below are correct)
a) Serves as a medium for transporting nutrients to, and wastes from, cells.
b) Serves as a medium to transport hormones, enzymes, platelets and red and white blood cells.
c) Important for cellular metabolism and proper cellular chemical functioning.
d) Helps maintain normal body temperature.
e) Solvent for electrolytes and nonelectrolytes.
f) Helps digestion and promotes elimination.
g) Necessary for the manufacture of body secretions.

6. Na+
7. Ca+
8. Cl-
9. HCO_3
10. K+
11. Ca+
12. Cl-
13. Na+
14. PO_4-

Organs of Homeostasis

15. A
16. F
17. B
18. D
19. C
20. E

Acid-Base Completion

21. phosphate, acid, alkaline
22. carbonic acid
23. ammonia, ammonium chloride
24. bicarbonate , H+
25. respiratory, carbonic acid, lungs
26 metabolic, bicarbonate, kidneys

Acid-Base Balance

27. metabolic alkalosis, carbon dioxide, K+, Na+, bicarbonate, H+, carbonic acid
28. respiratory alkalosis, hypoventilation, bicarbonate , H+
29. respiratory acidosis, carbon dioxide, bicarbonate, ammonium
30. metabolic acidosis, carbon dioxide, bicarbonate, H+

Nursing Implications of IV Therapy: Match

31. F
32. A
32. D, F
34. C
35. G
36. A,B,F
37. B
38. B,C
39. D
40. B,F

Unit VIII: Promoting Healthy Psychosocial Responses

Chapter 36: Self-Concept

Assessment Data/Key Terms Match

1. V
2. S
3. SS or C
4. SA or C
5. C
6. DM
7. P
8. IS
9. BI

Self-Concept Achievement

10. 3
11. 6
12. 5
13. 2
14. 4
15. 1

Chapter 37: Sensory Stimulation

Sensory Status: Match

1. B
2. C
3. D
4. A
5. E
6. A
7. B
8. D
9. C
10. E

Impaired Senses: Matching

11. H
12. S-T
13. V
14. S-T
15. T
16. V

Chapter 38: Sexuality

Search-a-Word

1. AIDS
2. BSE
3. cervix

4. penetration
5. cunnilingus
6. dyspareunia
7. ejaculation
9. erection
10. fellatio
11. fetishism
12. foreplay
13. gay
14. impotence
15. Kegel
16. lesbian
17. menarche
18. masochism
19. menapuase
20. menses
21. orgasm
22. ovulation
23. PID
24. sadism
25. sadomasochism
26. semen
27. sodomy
28. sexuality
29. sperm
30. STD
31. testes
32. uterus
33. vagina

Short Answer

34. The nurse should convey security and ease. Privacy, a relaxed atmosphere, an objective attitude on the part of the nurse, and confidentiality are important.
35. Beginning with non-threatening questions and progressing to more sensitive questions is a good way to start. Clients should understand why nurses need the information: to identify problems/concerns and to plan care. Using open-ended questions and a relaxed, non-judgmental approach is helpful.
36. a) Has anything interfered with your being a husband or father/wife or mother? b) Has anything changed the way you feel about yourself as a man/woman? c) Has anything changed your ability to function sexually?
37. The client needs to know what will happen to the information he gives and who will have access to it. He should be told that no one will have access to the information unless it is significant to his case.
38. Sexual desire is related to causative factors. A thorough assessment of causative factors is critical. Intervention should focus on modifying or controlling the causative factor(s), openly discussing problems/needed action with the partner, and planning time for relaxing/stroking/cuddling with the partner.
39. a) Assess past use and satisfaction/effectiveness, current knowledge of contraceptives and motivation to use contraceptives; b) Establish goals with client concerning use; c) Teach as needed; d) Evaluate achievement of client goals.
40. *Females*
    Date of menarche
    Date of last menstrual period
    Duration and length of flow
    Number of pregnancies, etc.
    Method of birth control used
    Known STDs, past or present
    Males
    Description of urinary function
    Number of children fathered
    Method of birth control used
    Know STDs, past or present
41. A model for counseling clients with sexual problems:
    P -- Permission giving
    LI -- Limited information
    SS -- Specific suggestions
    IT -- Intensive therapy

Chapter 39: Spirituality

Spirituality: True-False

1. False -- in ancient cultures
2. True
3. False -- can, sometimes
4. False, still have
5. True
6. False -- male Jewish infants
7. True
8. True
9. True
10. False -- accepted by some

Spirituality: Completion

11. blood transfusions
12. helpless
13. punishment, sin
14. religious ceremony
15. Reform, Conservative and Orthodox
16. Orthodox, Reform
17. Sabbath and Holy Days
18. Rabbi, confession
19. reconciliation
20. Holy Communion

Spirituality: Matching

21. D
22. A
23. B
24. E
25. C

Spirituality: Matching

26. D
27. E
28. G
29. A
30. C

(B & F are extra and match with nothing)

Crossword Puzzle

Across

3. agnostic
5. spirit
7. health
8. God
9. belief
11. grief
12. spirituality
18. value
20. ethnic
22. loss
26. anger
28. sin
29. distress
30. pain
31. religion

Down

1. alienate
2. mind
3. atheist
4. care
6. faith
9. body
10. forgive
13. priest
14. illness
15. love
16. needs
17. peace
19. joy
21. client
23. nursing
24. family
25. guilt
27. pray

Unit IX: Promoting Optimal Health in Special Situations

Chapter 40: Medications

Key Terms: Match

1. O
2. B
3. L
4. A
5. I
6. P
7. K
8. M
9. J
10. D
11. C
12. Q
13. F
14. H
15. G
16. E
17. N

Med Abbreviation Jeopardy

18. left eye
19. right eye
20. each eye
21. keep vein open
22. IV piggyback
23. discontinue
24. at bedtime; hour of sleep
25. intramuscular
26. intravenous
27. after meals
28. before meals
29. as desired
30. water
31. ointment
32. 3 times daily
33. suppository
34. every day
35. every hour
36. 4 times a day
37. every other day
38. take
39. subcutaneous
40. suspension
41. of each
42. twice a day
43. with
44. capsule
45. elixir
46. by mouth
47. by
48. as needed, when necessary
49. quantity sufficient
50. immediately
51. tincture

Calculating Medication Dosages
52. 1.5 cc
53. tab i
54. 0.5 tab
55. 3 tabs
56. 0.5 tab
57. 3 tabs
58. 0.25 tab (1/4 tab)
59. 0.5 tab (1/2 tab)
60. 2 tabs
61. 0.4 cc

Drug Preparations: Definitions
62. *capsule*: powder or gel form of an active drug enclosed in a gelatinous container
63. *elixir*: medication in a clear liquid containing water, alcohol, sweeteners, and flavor
64. *liniment*: medication mixed with alcohol, oil, or soap which is rubbed on the skin
65. *lotion*: drug particles in a solution for topical use
66. *lozenge*: small, oval, round or oblong preparation containing a drug in a flavored or sweetened base, which dissolves in the mouth releasing the medication
67. *ointment*: semisolid preparation containing a drug to be applied externally
68. *pill*: mixture of a powdered drug with a cohesive material; may be round or oval
69. *solution*: a drug dissolved in another substance
70. *suppository*: an easily melted medicated preparation in a firm base, such as gelatin, that is inserted into the body
71. *suspension*: finely divided, undissolved particles in a liquid medium
72. *syrup*: medication combined in a water and sugar solution
73. *tablet*: small, solid dosage of medication, compressed or molded

Common Abbreviations for Measures
74. *dram*: ʒ
75. *drops*: gtts
76. *grain*: gr
77. *milligram*: mg
78. *milliliter*: ml
79. *minim*: m or min
80. *ounce*: oz or ℥
81. *tablespoon* tbsp
82. *teaspoon*: tsp

Medication Procedures
83. The heparin lock, which is anchored in place to permit movement of the client, is flushed with a dilute heparin solution to check for intravenous placement and patency. To flush, the nurse aspirates then injects 1 ml solution. The medication is infused and the needle is replaced. The heparin lock is again flushed to clear the vein of medication. Finally, 1 ml of heparinized saline is injected to prevent clot formation.
84. IV piggyback is used for intermittent administration of a medication through an IV. The medication is mixed and hung by connecting the piggyback to the main intravenous line at the injection port. The main IV is lowered while the piggyback infuses. When the piggyback solution is infused, it is clamped off and the main IV is adjusted to its usual rate.

Chapter 41: Diagnostic Procedures

Diagnostic Procedures: Paragraph Completion
1. a) obtaining the consent; b) scheduling; c) physically; d) emotionally; e) comfort; f) equipment; g) specimen
2. a) sequence; b) barium enema; c) following; d) intravenous pyelogram; e) visualization
3. a) liver biopsy; b) right; c) insertion site; d) hemorrhage
4. a) Queckenstedt; b) jugular veins; c) increase; d) normal; e) blockage; f) prevent;) rising
5. a) during; b) following; c) color; d) pulse rate; e) respirations; f) fainting; g) nausea; h) vomiting; i) respiratory distress; j) punctured; k) severe coughing; l) bloody
6. a) electroencephalography; b) epilepsy; c) cerebrovascular; d) not; e) pain; f) discomfort; g) scalp; h) brain death

Diagnostic Exam: Matching
7. D
8. F
9. A
10. J
11. B
12. K
13. G
14. E
15. F
16. C
17. H
18. I
19. D
20. B
21. G
22. H

Nursing Interventions: Timeframe
23. C
24. A
25. C
26. B,C
27. B,C

28. C
29. A
30. A
31. B
32. A
33. A,B,C
34. C

Diagnostic Test Identification

35. colonoscopy
36. bronchoscopy
37. barium enema
38. cholecystogram
39. esophagogastroduodenoscopy or gastroscopy
40. intravenous pyelogram
41. cystoscopy
42. upper GI series
43. proctosigmoidoscopy
44. a fasting blood sugar

Diagnostic Tests Commonalities

45. both tests involve the use of barium
46. both are painless and both require the use of electrodes
47. both are for the purpose of fluid withdrawal and can result in the puncture of an organ
48. both require that the client be in a fasting state
49. client must maintain a prescribed position for the test
50. neither test requires any special preparation

Nursing Diagnoses

51-53.

Potential complication of invasive diagostic procedure (liver biopsy, paracentesis, etc): hemorrhage, respiratory distress, etc.

a. Knowledge deficit regarding ordered diagnostic test or procedure

b. Anxiety related to inexperience or lack of knowledge regarding ordered diagnostic examination

c. Knowledge deficit regarding preparation for diagnostic test

d. Knowledge deficit regarding restrictions required following diagnostic test/procedure

e. Fear related to results of diagnostic test for (cancer, liver disease, heart disease, etc.)

Chapter 42: Care of Wounds

Wound Types

1. B
2. B
3. A
4. B
5. A
6. A
7. A
8. B
9. B
10. B
11. A
12. B
13. A
14. A
15. B
16. A

Wound Descriptors

17. contusion; hard; closed; blood vessels; swelling; pain; internal organs
18. intentional; asepsis; instrument; needle
19. puncture; penetrates; skin; tissues; intentional
20. jagged; laceration; trauma; unclean; infection
21. abrasion; scrape; intentional

Wound Characteristics: Matching

22. B
23. A
24. D
25. C
26. A
27. B
28. C
29. C
30. D
31. A

Word Scramble

32. approximation
33. bandage
34. binder
35. cold
36. contusion
37. debridement
38. dressing
39. wet
40. evisceration
41. exudate
42. granulation
43. heat
44. hemorrhagic
45. incision
46. moist
47. pack
48 puncture
49. purulent
50. retention sutures
51. sanguineous
52. scar
53. scultetus binder
54. serous
55. skin
56. stab wound
57. trauma

58. dry
59. wound

Surgical Drains

60. J-P
61. gauze drains
62. penrose
63. hemovac
64. T-tube

Wound Care: True/False

65. True
66. False: acetate is used for small wounds and to secure dressings
67. True
68. False: decreased urinary output
69. True
70. True
71. False: she documents each time wound care is given
72. False: they require changing only as necessary, ie: when soiled
73. True
74. True

Nursing Actions in Wound Care

75. Controls temperature and extends therapeutic effect of compress
76. Hot water bottle molds more easily to area and puts less pressure on site. Air reduces pliability of bag.
77. Cotton tip of applicator absorbs wound drainage
78. Irrigation removes exudate and debris
79. To clean from least to most contaminated area

Nursing Diagnoses/Interventions

80. a) Encourage client to express fears regarding performance of home wound care/dressing changes; b) Answer all questions; c) Teach client/SO to thoroughly wash hands prior to and after care; d) Teach client/SO wound care/dressing change; e) Have client perform return demonstration for correct procedure
81. a) Perform sterile dressing changes; b) Assess wound for appearance and drainage; c) Monitor temperature, pulse and respirations; d) Culture wound as ordered
82. a) Teach client to splint abdomen when coughing; b) Teach client relaxation techniques to reduce pain and increase effectiveness of pain medications; c) Encourage ambulation/activity as ordered; d) Encourage client to request pain medications before pain is severe

Chapter 43: Perioperative Care

Surgery Classification

1. C
2. A
3. C
4. B
5. A
6. B
7. A
8. A
9. B
10. A
11. B
12. E
13. C
14. F
15. A
16. D
17. B
18. C
19. D
20. A
21. F

Levels of Anesthesia

22. warmth, detachment, numbness, dizziness; client is conscious
23. uncontrolled movement, struggling, talking, laughing; client is conscious
24. no feelings or expressions; client is unconscious
25. no feelings or expressions; emergency situation of respiratory arrest and vasomotor collapse; client is unconscious and can die

Local and Regional Anesthesia

26. subarachnoid space; for surgery of lower abdomen and below; hypotension, headache or urinary retention
27. used on mucus membranes, skin, wound and burns
28. injected around nerve trunk; used for jaw, face, extremities
29. injected into tissues; used for biopsies and skin suturing

Perioperative True/False

30. False - agree by signing an informed consent form
31. False - preoperative assessment and teaching are essential elements in safe surgery and recovery
32. True
33. False - identifies physical and psychosocial risk factors and strengths
34. True
35. True
36. True
37. False - ambulatory surgery is no different from inpatient surgery in this respect; a cold or infection may necessitate cancelling of surgery
38. False - teaching is done regarding the surgery during the preoperative period
39. True

Client Goals

40. Client will be able to verbalize purpose of surgery and events to occur OR Client will be emotionally prepared for surgery.
41. Client will demonstrate correctly, how to turn, cough, deep breathe, and splint the incision
42. Client will maintain symmetric breathing patterns throughout surgery
43. Client will be free of infection from wound contamination
44. Client will deep-breathe and cough effectively every 2 hours as taught OR Client will remain free of respiratory complications
45. Client will have a balanced intake and output
46. Client will verbalize decreasing pain on a scale of 1 to 10
47. Client will correctly demonstrate wound care and dressing changes

Postoperative Complications

48. thrombophlebitis - inflammation of a vein associated with blood clot formation
49. pneumonia - inflammation of the alveoli due to an infectious process or foreign material
50. hemorrhage - excessive blood loss, either internally or externally
51. shock - acute peripheral circulatory failure due to loss of circulatory control or circulating fluid
52. atelectasis - incomplete expansion or collapse of alveoli due to retained mucus
53. paralytic ileus - absence of peristalsis
54. pulmonary embolus - an embolus lodged in the pulmonary vessels
55. evisceration - viscera protruding through an incision postoperatively

Drugs and Surgical Risks

56. tranquilizers
57. anticoagulants
58. adrenal steroids
59. the "mycin" antibiotics
60. diuretics

Nursing Interventions: Matching

61. B
62. C
63. E
64. A
65. F
66. D
67. C
68. A
69. B
70. D,C
71. E,D

Rationale for Nursing Actions

72. promotes wound healing
73. minimizes surgical risk and reduces client anxiety regarding postoperative period
74. decreases potential for infection by reducing number of microorganisms on skin
75. minimizes risk of injury or complications during or after surgery
76. cuts may be a potential source of infection
77. decreased body temperature results from depressed level of functioning
78. blood may drain beneath client. Hemorrhage & shock are life threatening surgical complications
79. anesthetic agents depress respiratory functions. Turning promotes respiratory function until client can be ambulatory
80. anesthetics depress peristalsis and normal GI functioning
81. edema may indicate complication such thrombophlebitis, emboli, or congestive heart failure
82. indicates potential respiratory complications such as pneumonia or atelectasis
83. provides baseline data for intra- and postoperative phases

Surgical Risks in the Elderly

84. *Renal*: reduced bladder capacity; decreased renal blood flow
85. *Respiratory:* diminished cough reflex; reduced vital capacity; decreased oxygenation of blood
86. *Cardiovascular:* decreased cardiac output, reserve and heart rate; decreased peripheral circulation; increased vascular rigidity
87. *Integument:* dry, inelastic skin; decreased vascularity
88. *Neurologic:* decreased reaction time; sensory deficit